Ohhmazing Wellness

SHIFT YOUR VISION AND CREATE THE HEALTHY & HAPPY LIFESTYLE YOU DESERVE!

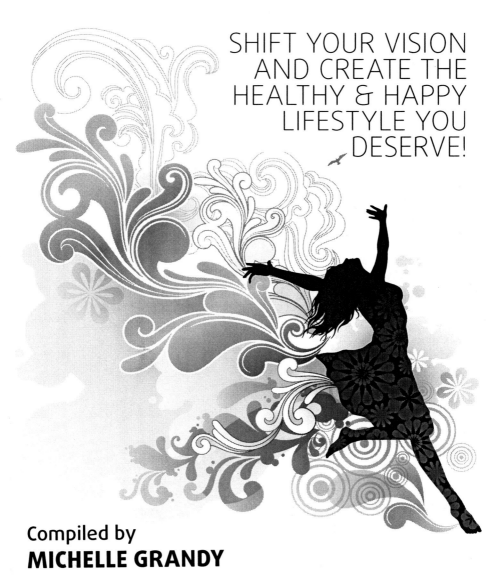

Compiled by
MICHELLE GRANDY

CM Publisher
c/o Marketing for Coach, Ltd
Second Floor
6th London Street
W2 1HR London (UK)

www.cm-publisher.com
info@cm-publisher.com

ISBN: 978-0-9929876-3-3

Published in UK, Europe, US and Canada

Book Cover: Csernik Előd

Inside Layout: Csernik Előd

Table of Contents

Gratitude

It was an absolute pleasure to work alongside the lovely co-authors of *Ohhmazing Wellness: Shift Your Vision and Create the Healthy & Happy Lifestyle You Deserve!* I have a deep-rooted sense of gratitude knowing these co-authors used their instincts to give of themselves and share their stories, tips, and resources in this book. I would like to thank all the professional co-authors for accepting my invitation and saying *YES* to collectively collaborate on this book about integrative wellness. You all are beautiful, powerful, and courageous women and your spirit, love, dedication, and voices during this entire engaging process was an *Ohhmazing* journey for me and I pray the same for you. I will always be grateful. With all of us working and living busy lives, I am grateful we found time to support and encourage each other as we worked to meet deadline after deadline and accomplish the goal of writing our stories. I would not have been able to make this book happen without the diverse stories from each of you.

I give honor to God and am thankful to Him for instilling the vision in me to move forward on this anthology book project, and for identifying thirty women from across the world to collaborate on this effort. It was because of God's grace and my faithfulness that I was able to bring together thirty women to share their wellness wisdom to inspire, empower, and encourage a generation of women to step out of their comfort zones and into something new and powerful. What a powerful God we serve!

I want to thank my family: my *Ohhmazing* and wise husband, Albert; my four incredibly awesome and wise sons: Jamal, Albert III, Michael and Wayne; and my brother, Michael, for your awareness, your love and allowing me space to work at all times of the day and night in collaborating the efforts of this book. Thank you for the daily inspiration, love, and support you give me. I am truly blessed to have you and grateful to be called your wife, mom, and sister. I want to thank my family and friends for their continuous faith and believing that if anyone could get this book accomplished, it would be me. Thank you for allowing me to call, text, and email you when I needed to hear your voice during late nights and very early mornings. I would like to thank my social media friends and family for showing love with likes, comments, and sharing during the endless posting about this book.

I want to thank Canyon Ranch and the Canyon Ranch Institute family, Charles and Rosalie Morris, and Curtis V. Cooper Primary Health Care for the life transforming experience which lead me to selecting the title of this book on integrative wellness. It was my eleven-day stay at Canyon Ranch, Tuscon, AZ in December 2013 where I received my inspiration to write about self-care as it relates to eight areas of a woman's life. The knowledge, information, experiences, and connection with Canyon Ranch and Canyon Ranch Institute community left me empowered and inspired to help change the way women think about wellness as it relates to taking care of our total wellbeing.

Introduction

What do the words *take care of yourself* actually mean to you? Can I assume you say these words but often do not find time to actually put the words in action? What does "self-care" mean to you and why is it important? Are you so busy taking care of others you neglect your self-care needs? Do you agree that if you don't take care of yourself then you are the one who truly suffers in the end? Do you agree that the following are relevant areas of self-care?

- Spa and Beauty
- Food and Nutrition
- Fitness and Movement
- Health and Holistic Healing
- Mind and Spirit
- Relationships
- Career and Entrepreneurship
- Finances

Do you long for more time to work on any of these self-care areas?

As women, way too often we neglect to feed our body, mind, and soul with what it really needs to be present, authentically vibrant, and whole. There is no better time to get realistic with practical ways to engage in the act of self-love than by reading and hearing the stories from the co-authors in this book. *Ohhmazing Wellness: Shift Your Vision and Create the Healthy & Happy Lifestyle You Deserve* is a collaboration voiced in print of thirty beautiful, powerful, and courageous women from across the world who share their personal and authentic stories to empower women everywhere to believe in acts of wellness through self-care. These courageous women take you on a journey through their lives—revealing their struggles, despair, boldness, and triumph. They bring you to an inspired space of living a healthy and happy lifestyle through love, truth and acceptance. These stories are about stepping out of your comfort zone, healthy new beginnings, breaking down walls, living with what is, transformation and possibilities, loving food, listening to your body and trusting your body, and embracing the change, and much more. You will be inspired to connect with the woman you are on the inside, indulge in self-care like never before, and create the life you dream and deserve. The good news is that these *Ohhmazing* women are just like us, as we are busy with family, careers, running businesses, taking care of our parents, volunteering, coaching, teaching, and being life-long students. So I ask you again, what do the words *take care of yourself* mean to you? Allow the stories in this book to help bring forth your powerful answer!

Each chapter is an absolute gem, a source of *Ohhmazing* inspiration, and a meaningful moment of truth. This book is the only tool you'll ever need to step onto the path towards your own success with wellness, confidence, and self-belief. It is written with love and authenticity.

I encourage you to find a quiet space, as you will be utterly surprised over what is revealed inside this book!

Most of us have a book that changed our life...this book will not only cause you to shift your vision around wellness and self-care, it will also ensure you reach success through wellness in the areas of self-care within your life. Here's to shifting your vision to create the healthy and happy lifestyle you deserve! Namaste.

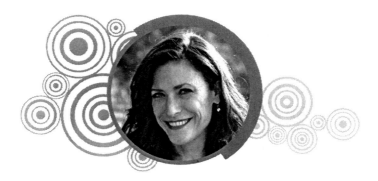

Debra Zadoorian, RYT

As a martial artist, certified Baptist-inspired yoga teacher, photographer, and master stylist and color expert, Debra brings a unique perspective on what constitutes authentic beauty. She approaches beauty by incorporating inner-peace, self-awareness, and spirituality so that together they radiate physically, mentally, and emotionally.

Debra owns Tola Hair Studio and her formal training extends over twenty-five years. She's pursued her passion for authentic beauty throughout her adult life. Her mastery of wide-ranging authentic beauty techniques has kept her at the forefront of her field and makes her uniquely qualified as a contributing author.

www.tolahairstudio.com

 debra@tolahairstudio.com

CHAPTER 1

BEAUTY WITH BENEFITS

By Debra Zadoorian, RYT

As a child, let's just say I looked at myself in the mirror and thought, *YUCK!!!* I hated my hair, puffy circles under my eyes, and big nose. So I decided if I didn't look in the mirror, maybe I could pretend I wasn't ugly. On top of that, I was known as the kid who lived in the shack. My house was made fun of just about every day. It was hurtful and embarrassing, especially because I never knew who was going to join in. The girls I thought were my friends were just as bad as the boys. I was convinced I was the ugly girl who lived in the ugly house. Interestingly, I never told my parents any of this—I guess I thought I was protecting them. They kept me balanced through the bullying, even though they were unaware of what I was going through. The love and confidence showered by my parents taught me that beauty is so much more than the vision in the mirror. I was able to see individuals for whom and what they were and where they were coming from. I was able to sympathize and empathize with anyone. I feel so blessed to see a beauty in people that they don't tend to see in themselves. I am so grateful for each and every day I have ever had and look forward to the life I will have. Beauty comes from within. No matter what a person has been blessed with or without, it's the light from the heart that brings sunshine to the hearts that are dimmed.

Living healthy decisions by eating a healthy diet, taking vitamins, drinking sufficient amounts of water, and doing yoga, exercise, and meditation is all vital to creating and sustaining authentic beauty. I believe adding yoga to your routine can only enhance your life. The body is like a garden and will respond beautifully when it is properly fed. Skin becomes hydrated, nails become stronger, hair responds by shining and growing faster. The eyes clearly sparkle and you look and feel healthier.

Sometimes we want to do the right things for ourselves but we don't think we have the time, or maybe we need to be inspired. One way to jump start yourself into a new way of being is to go to a reputable spa and treat yourself to a massage, facial, manicure, pedicure, waxing, scalp treatments, and possibly a new hairstyle or color. If you're unable to have all of this at the same time, start with the massage. This will set the tone in your body, mind, and spirit.

There are many different types of massage. Swedish, deep tissue, hot stone, Thai, and pregnancy massage, just to name a few. If you are unfamiliar to massage, do a little research to determine the style that may be right for you and ask around to find some recommendations on a licensed massage therapist who specializes in the style you choose. A great massage does so many things. It helps to break up those tight knots of pent-up stress, it relaxes your body and mind, creates a better blood flow to areas that are tight, and helps to create an inner peace.

The pedicure and manicure need to be completed by a licensed technician. I know this may seem obvious, but you would be surprised with what is out there. It is so important that your services are completed with instruments that are properly sanitized. Bacteria and fungus can easily move from one person to the next on nail utensils that haven't been properly sterilized. Bringing your own tools will eliminate that risk. Even in the most pristine salons, these tools may not be replaced after each customer. Also, a fresh liner should be in the pedicure tub and the water aerator needs to be sanitized after each client. Lastly, make sure that their pedicure chair has a pipeless jet system. If not, I would suggest another salon with updated chairs. There is no way for you to know if proper sanitation has been performed. According to the American Academy of Dermatology, pedicure health risks include fungal infections, such as athlete's foot and nail fungus, and bacterial skin infections, including MRSA (Methicillin-resistant Staphylococcus aureus), a potentially serious antibiotic-resistant staph infection. The Centers for Disease Control and Prevention and the Environmental Protection Agency warn against shaving, using hair removal creams, or waxing your legs and feet during the twenty-four hours before getting a pedicure. Hair removal can cause cuts or subtle abrasions that you would not notice on your feet. The smallest opening in the skin can allow fungus and bacteria to enter.

Facials are beneficial for so many reasons. A facial cleans, exfoliates, and nourishes the skin, promoting a well-hydrated clear complexion and can create a younger, healthier, and glowing appearance. There are many different types of facials on the market right now. Again, it's doing a research on what's available and having a great recommendation. The esthetician is also a resource for educating you on taking care of your skin with a daily regimen and possibly prescribing a skin care line that will benefit and protect your skin between facial appointments.

There are many different treatments being used for the removal of unwanted body hair: waxing, laser, and electrolysis are a few of the more popular methods. I suggest that keeping up with your eyebrows is a great asset. When having your eyebrows shaped, you want to keep them as natural as possible. Have an arch created or maintained without thinning the brow down too much. If your eyebrows are light or thin, have your hairdresser darken them to match your hair color. Daily maintenance can be obtained with an eyebrow pencil or gel. That being said, keep the pressure light and keep the natural appearance. These enhancements will bring more focus to your eyes.

When you apply your makeup, keep in mind you only want to enhance your beauty. Some people use their face as a blank canvas and create their version of who they think they should be. When you look in the mirror, start by looking at yourself knowing you already are beautiful. Your makeup is just a tool to hide areas you are not happy with and enhancing what we are proud of. If you're not familiar with how to apply makeup and need some help, you could hire a makeup artist to teach you or simply search the web for technical videos. As Zoë Zadoorian mentions in her chapter, YouTube is a great source of helpful information.

Your hair and scalp are things you need to pamper. You want to keep them healthy so your hair will grow luxuriously. Scalp treatments, conditioning treatments, and great quality hair products are essential. Finding a great hairdresser that is licensed and experienced is as important as finding a great doctor. You want someone who believes it is essential to keep the integrity of the hair. This speaks loudly to hair colorists. You want to go to someone who is able to color your hair without compromising the condition of your hair or scalp. If your hair doesn't feel better after a chemical service, you need a better hairdresser/colorist. Stylists have been known to save money by using low-quality products or by scrimping on products. For instance, if you're having your gray roots covered, are they glossing your ends with a hydrating gloss or are they leaving the ends bare? Or worse, are they running the same color down the shaft at any point of the service? Hmm, you deserve better. Luxurious hair color, highlight, lowlight or customized hair painting, and body waves are just a few techniques that may be incorporated with a customized haircut/style.

I am the proud owner of Tola Hair Studio in Bluffton, South Carolina. I have clients come to me every day so I can help them maintain or renew their appearance. Feeling beautiful and confident is something we all strive for in one way or another. The secret to our success is by honing into a *healthy* beautiful and keeping an open heart. Let's face it, when we feel good, we look better. When we live good, we love better. We create an authentic happiness that brings an inner peace and outstanding beauty.

Lastly, doing our best to manage our stress levels is so important to our overall beauty. When we are over-stressed, we start to lose focus. When we lose focus, we begin to spin out of control. Exercising, eating healthy, and other positive things begin to take the backseat to priority. Try to incorporate meditation and yoga to your daily routine. There are many opportunities at home with YouTube videos, podcasts, or in your community at a local yoga studio. Through my yoga and meditation, I have been able to find an inner peace that helps me stay focused on what is really important—being present to myself and to others without being mentally cluttered. Namaste.

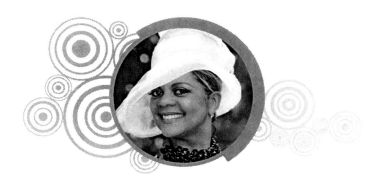

Vernell Washington, CEO

No matter what your destination—from Paris to Peru, a show-stopping hat assures you'll be arriving in style, according to globetrotting Vernell Washington—CEO of Grand Diva Enterprises. As she should know, always smartly clad in boldly hued apparel, with sexy silhouettes, typically accessorized with a flamboyant hat.

The Philadelphia native graduated from the famed Fashion Institute of Technology (FIT) in NY. This sealed her life's path as the ultimate fashionista. While traveling the world to find the "best of the best," she found herself in Lagos, Nigeria, the ultimate fashion capital of the world. Her fun loving, enthusiastic personality caught the attention of Grace Mark—one of Africa's most renowned milliners. Mark saw the dazzling diva as the key to opening doors in the United States and beyond.

Their mutual respect for creativity, craftsmanship, and a love for chic couture chapeau, this duo created a wonderful partnership between Grace's Hats and Grand Diva Enterprises. To view the latest "one of a kind" hat collections, media, magazine, and newspaper articles, visit: www.granddivaenterprises.com.

✉ **Vernelll@granddivaentrprises.com**
🅕 **Vernell Granddiva Washington**
🅧 **Granddiva100**
🅞 **Granddiva100**

11

CHAPTER 2

HATS BRING HAPPINESS

By Vernell Washington, CEO

As we journey through life searching our minds, bodies and souls for the PERFCT answer to happiness, I would like to interject what actually completes the total package of "self worth", self being and infinite happiness. We all know that whoever we are, we want to have a since of belonging, a since of being loved and in return, giving back the best love that your mind and spirit can give. That uplift in the spirit happens simply by someone complimenting you on the way you look. This simple, kind gesture turn a sad gloomy day into a day filled with brightness and joy. SELF ESTEEM is the key element that enables us to walk up tall, strut our stuff, put a little glide in our stride and simply take on the world with confidence. When you wake up in the morning and do your daily ritual of washing your face, brushing your teeth, putting on your make-up, doing your hair,putting the right outfit on, the perfect pumps, the brightest lipstick and heading out the door to conquer the world with confidence, you find that the world gives you the nod of acceptance by smiling back at you as you glide and glisten through the day. They are acknowledging your outer beauty, your inner glow and the self confidence that exudes because you are looking good and feeling good. Feeling good because you have gotten the acceptance from the outside world that you are beautiful.

I always knew that there was a connection between "outward beauty" and self- esteem. That is why I decided to fulfill my passion for fashion by getting into the fashion industry. I was born and raised in The City of Brotherly Love. My hometown which is a stone throw from the Fashion Capital of the World…New York City! I have always been daring in my fashion forward choices in clothing. I would have fun mixing stripes and polka dots, leopard and cow print and just an array of combinations. Then I would always wear my hair back and throw on my signature scarf, tied in a bow on the back of my ponytail. Oh, did I say….add the bold jewelry and then of course, the brightest orange or pink lipstick that I could find. After putting all of my garb on, I was ready to "take on the world". As I approached the world, the big blue sunny skies, illuminating the outdoors, I realized that I not only made myself happy by being bright, colorful and "outside the box" with my style, I noticed that it always made others happy by appreciating my fashion sense. As I would strut down the street, holding my head up high, I received lots of smiles, compliments and infectious nods. It also afforded me the opportunity to receive special treatment. When I would walk into a store, restaurant, hotel, bar or club, they would always place me up front, allow me to enter first or offer me complimentary things. All of this wonderful special treatment, compliments, feedback, praise and warm welcoming has helped to mold my inner self worth, my inner happiness, and has given me the strength to carry on in life as a positive, loving, giving, content, human being.

Since Fashion was my passion, I decided to build upon my unique, expressive fashion sense, and move to New York City to attend the top fashion school in the world. Fashion Institute of Technology F.I.T. After getting my dual degrees in Fashion Buying and Merchandising and in Production Management, I was off to the races! The sky was the limit for me. In New York City, I had a flourishing modeling career, retail clothing career, jewelry and accessories business and furrier business. I thoroughly enjoyed all of those careers and I still incorporate all of those elements as part of my brand.

The BRAND….. One day, my dear friend Helen had a DIVA luncheon at the Four Seasons in Atlanta. She had just attended an Oprah Winfrey convention which really inspired her about life, love, friendships, happiness, and connections with ladies. At this Diva event, we were all required to wear our best "fashionista" attire and to wear a hat. I arrived 10 minutes early, but another friend caught me before I got on the elevator to ask me to wait for her so that we could go upstairs together. Since I waited for her, we ended up being about 1 minute late. After getting off of the elevator, we ran up the hall, with shopping bags in our hands, ran into the lovely place set tables, with all of the ladies sitting around in their beautiful attire. I remember wearing a cream colored ensemble with a baaaaad hat on. As I ran into the room, one girl blurted out…here she comes….that's The Grand Diva! I chuckled but the name has stuck with me ever since. I have created my ultimate fashion business under the name of Grand Diva Enterprises. My company has helped many people make lifestyle changes. We have transformed many women from ordinary to extraordinary by outfitting them with the latest, innovative trends. Whether it be the latest clothing trend or the boldest jewelry and accessories or hat.

So that I stay on top of the latest and greatest in fashion trends and forecasts, I usually attend several fashion shows each year. Around 2001 I attended a big fashion show sponsored by the United Nations. They utilized the Atlanta Falcon Cheerleaders to model in the show. Can I tell you that it was one of the best shows that I had attended, mainly because the show highlighted one of the most brilliant milliners in the world! Grace Mark, came all the way from Lagos Nigeria to show her "one of a kind" masterpieces in the fashion extravaganza event. My jaw dropped in awe of Grace's creations as each model walked out with a blazingly awesome chapeaux.

I walked up to her after the show and told her how talented she was and that I HAD to represent her in the states. There was no ifs ands or buts about it. I told her, that her hats had to be shown for the world to see. She agreed and we hit the ground running. Our partnership was born! Under the name of Grand Diva Enterprises. I am the Global Representative for Grace's Hats. And Global Representative it is! Grace's hats are in London, Dubai, Paris, Bermuda, Canada, Bahamas, St. Lucia and all across the United States and the Globe. We have been on several talk shows, and have been featured in various newspaper and magazine in the U.S., Africa, London and the Associated Press. Most importantly, Grace's hats win awards for the "Best Hat", virtually every hat contest that her hats are entered into. The Kentucky Derby, The London Ascots and The Atlanta Steeple Chase just to name a few.

We are even a member of The Hat Ladies of Charleston, which is a group of hat wearing ladies that participate in lots of charitable events.

They donate their time, energy and happiness that they bring to others, because they wear their hats to help others. Each year we host a dynamic luncheon in NY called The Hats of the World Luncheon (H.O.W.L) which is attended by many of the lady Ambassadors of the World. It is held at the United Nations.

Just as I enjoyed looking at women in hats, so do others. Men in particular, marvel over the mere sight of a woman wearing a beautiful hat! It has been the African American tradition for hundreds of years to "wear a crown" to church. I have found a few clichés from the" Crowns" book very interesting.

"Countless black women would rather attend church naked than hatless".

"A church hat as flamboyant as it may be, it is no mere fashion accessory. It's a cherished African American custom."

"A woman's hat speaks long before its wearer utters a word."

"There's a little more strut in your carriage when you wear a nice hat."

All of these sayings are the true sentiments of die hard hat lovers.

Jaqueline Kennedy Onassis brought the hat fashion trend to an all-time high in the 1960's and of course Lady Diana in London was smashing in her outfit and hat ensembles. She rattled the world and sent the paparazzi spinning in their tracks.

As we age gracefully, certain types of hats are great to wear in the sun so we can get the protection from the UV rays. The big floppy hats are great for that protection along with some huge Hollywood shades.

Hats can be worn to the beach, to church, for ladies night out, to luncheons, to weddings, funerals, cocktail sips, to the park and of course for bad hair days.

Wherever you are, whatever you do.....WEAR A HAT, BE HAPPY AND LET THE WHOLE WORLD KNOW IT!!!

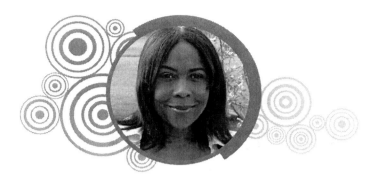

Y. Walton Davis, LE, MUA

Y. Walton Davis is a professional television and video makeup artist and stylist, licensed esthetician, beauty consultant, and writer.

A Chicago native, Y. Walton Davis is a graduate of communications from Columbia College Chicago. With over fourteen years of experience in broadcast media and the beauty industry, Y. has contributed to some of the most viewed programming around the world including The Oprah Winfrey Show, Oprah Radio, OWN, Fox News, and the NBA.

She's known for her "you, but better" approach to beauty in helping women look and feel their very best.

✉ **Jovetstudio@hotmail.com**

f **facebook.com/Jovetstudio**

f **facebook.com/Y.Walton Davis**

g+ **googleplus.com/Jovet studio**

in **linkedin.com/Jovet studio**

CHAPTER 3

THE BEAUTY
OF TRANSFORMING OURSELVES

By Y. Walton Davis, LE, MUA

Having a career in television as an image stylist and makeup artist, as well as a consultant and esthetician in the beauty industry, has tremendously helped me to reevaluate my views of what beauty really is and I've discovered that an internal makeover is the true and lasting essence of real beauty.

Being around so many illusions of what beauty was supposed to resemble, I quickly realized that I needed more than just an external representation of beauty in my life. Many of my experiences in my life and career—good and bad—have consistently challenged me to unlock my inner self in order to find a higher purpose and meaning in my journey. I'm a firm believer that women who are not in touch with their inner selves run the risk of living somewhat meaningless and unfulfilled lives.

We're conditioned as women to feel that we can "have it all," but often, with so many hats to juggle in our lives, we get overwhelmed and unfortunately lose ourselves in that process. The guilt of not meeting everyone's expectations can leave us feeling mentally exhausted and sometimes even depressed. I had to accept the fact that if I didn't make my well-being a priority, it would be difficult to create a balanced lifestyle for me and my family. Having the courage to transform and renew old ideas and patterns that keep us bound in comprising situations is the first step to building a healthier and happier life.

I'm amazed that so many women I meet express that they don't have enough time to nurture themselves properly. I explain to them I was once in their shoes and truly understand their dilemma of feeling overwhelmed with so many facets of just being a woman. I encourage these women to count the cost of neglecting themselves and I help them to see the benefits of self-care and give them simple solutions that can be incorporated into their daily routines.

Like so many families growing up, as a teenager I observed the women in my family who would sacrifice themselves for the family, but I could see this would leave them feeling mentally, physically, and spiritually depleted trying to balance a household efficiently and trying to meet the never-ending demands of life.

My wakeup call came in 2002 when my mother was diagnosed with breast cancer. As soon as she told me, I felt devastated and I began to cry—not just for my mother but for all women who felt they had to neglect their own well-being to become the "super-woman" for everyone else. At that moment, I realized my mother had given so much to our family and forgotten about her own well-being. I knew I wanted to help change that pattern in my family so the next generation of women would be ready to conquer the world with more balanced ideas of self and the ability to truly understand the value of self-preservation. So I began researching and buying cosmetics and food brands that were committed to a healthier approach in creating their products. It's still one of my passions today to know how brands are formulated, especially when your loved one is going through a medical crisis. My mother's battle with breast cancer helped me to understand how women tend to put everyone's needs before their own, and I knew this cycle needed to be stopped in order for my family and I to live a more purposeful and meaningful life.

Despite this challenging time for my mom, I'm so grateful to say she is now living a life with more direction and making healthier choices combined with a balanced diet and exercise. I had always tried to eat healthy combined with exercise but I truly believe my mom's health challenge was instrumental in helping our entire family to make better lifestyle choices.

Becoming an esthetician allowed me to educate women on the benefits of facials, exfoliation, and many other spa therapies, and with a little effort, women could create a spa-like atmosphere in their own homes. My career choice was always with the intent to help improve and inspire women to look and feel better about themselves, so of course I started with myself and the women in my own family. I had researched products that would not only help us look better but products that would improve our overall well-being. I would invite my mom, sister, and nieces over for a pamper day that would sometimes be a facial day, salon day, or tea party day—suggested by one of my nieces who at the time was only seven years of age.

The tea party experience ended up being the most rewarding for me and allowed us to get closer and stronger as women, while sipping tea. We were so blessed that my niece could understand the benefits of coming together and sharing our experiences as females.

We all felt these gatherings were transforming all of our lives in a profound and loving way that none of us had ever experienced. We would laugh, cry, and sometimes debate, but at the end of the day we all realized the bond we shared as family—and women—could never be broken.

From the beginning of our first women gatherings, I realized these simple acts of getting together and enjoying a cup tea, or just indulging in a spa facial, were key components to us looking and feeling better about ourselves as women for the rest of our lives.

Developing all aspects of ourselves as women can be difficult, especially when we don't know how to balance the people in our relationships.

I spent so many years of my life trying to find my way in developing the whole woman, and yes, I would come up short in this area of my life. I'm the first to admit that I was guilty of the "people-pleasing syndrome," but at that time I had no idea this syndrome was not about the other person but me feeling insecure in myself as an individual and forgetting to honor myself first. I'm in no way suggesting it's all about ourselves as women, but it is essential for us to balance every aspect of our lives in order to give back in a more balanced manner.

There's an old saying that resonates in my mind and that is: "When we know better, we do better." And I am so proud to say my family and I are doing so much better and we are looking forward to a future that is filled with more balance and purpose.

Spending time with the women in my family gave me a better sense of who they were and opened up my heart to understand that we truly do need one another as women for friendship and support.

I'm a firm believer women function better when we take the time to nurture ourselves from the inside out, and with this mindset, we become more successful in all our endeavors and responsibilities in life.

My "internal nurturing" beauty secrets that I embrace when putting on my makeup before starting my day:

Internal beauty secrets:

- Foundation has the ability to cover all my imperfections on my face but it is a reminder I must not beat myself up for the flaws that need to be corrected in my life. Learning to be more patient with myself is the foundation to having better patience with everything in my life.

- Lipstick brings bold and beautiful colors to my mouth so I always want my mouth to speak words that heal and encourage.

- Blush is great for radiance and brightening my face, and a reminder to always bring sunshine, joy, and laughter to the world.

- Eye shadow colors can make my eyes look natural or more dramatic but my goal when I wear it is to see with less judgment and more love.

Being committed to transforming ourselves from the inside out and understanding the beauty of balancing our lives is what I believe leads us to the true foundation of creating lives filled with joy, happiness, and most of all love. Learning to listen and take action from internal signs we often ignore can help us advance and transform our overall well-being. Understanding the beauty of transforming our mind,

21

body, and spirit can lead us to treasures beyond our wildest dreams. The wellness days, especially the tea parties with the women in my family, gave all of us a place to free our minds, reflect on our lives, and rejoice in the fact that these simple pleasures motivated us to make positive changes, which caused a major shift of growth in our development as women. And I am happy to say this has been one of my great treasures in life that I was blessed to find and will cherish forever.

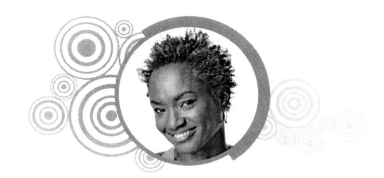

Michelle Grandy,
CHHC, AADP, RYT, CFCRI

Michelle is passionate about helping others change their thought process on health and wellness. As a wellness enthusiast, she is the founder/CEO of Ohh Michelle, LLC, a company dedicated to supporting and empowering people to reconnect with their body, mind, and soul through nutrition, yoga, and wellness. Her gift is empowerment and she uses her education and talents to usher busy individuals to make a lifestyle change. Michelle is a Certified Holistic Health Practitioner through the Institute of Integrative Nutrition, Registered Yoga Instructor through Yoga Alliance, Canyon Ranch Institute Certified Facilitator, Plant-Based Lifestyle Coach/Chef, Motivational Speaker and International Best Selling Author. Michelle has been married for 22 years, has four ohhmazing sons and resides in the Hilton Head, SC. area.

www.ohhmichelle.com

- facebook.com/OHHMICHELLEOM
- facebook.com/mtgrandy
- twitter.com/michelletgrandy
- instagram.com/ohhmichelle
- google.com/+MichelleGrandyOM
- youtube.com/user/Mtgrandy27

23

CHAPTER 4

STEP OUT OF YOUR COMFORT ZONE

By Michelle Grandy, CHHC, AADP, RYT, CFCRI

"Yoga is a journey into truth. Truth about who you really are.
What you are capable of and how your actions affect your
life. It all starts within your body and on your mat."

~ Baron Baptiste

I've learned that yoga is about breath and movement. We breathe in to inhale fresh air and we breathe out to release toxins. Our family had moved from Syracuse, NY, down to the Hilton Head, SC, area with a new job opportunity for my husband. It felt like we were a military family since we moved so much—and both of us are from the Washington, DC, area (I from NW Washington and my husband from Capitol Heights, MD). We moved from DC to Atlanta where we lived for eight years and from Atlanta to Upstate, NY, for seven years, and again from NY to the Low Country area. Moving down south was a time of getting the kids settled into the new environment, new home, and new school. It was also a fresh start for me, because the often dark and cold environment started to affect my emotional state. Therefore, I welcomed the move down south. I welcomed change!

The night before my forty-seventh birthday, I contemplated how I wanted to celebrate. I planned to wake up, give thanks and honor to God, and go take a yoga class. Yes, I was forty-seven years old when I first entered a yoga studio—a local yoga studio in Bluffton, SC. Reading the yoga class offerings didn't matter much because I was new to yoga and had no knowledge about the different types of yoga. Although I had heard of the studio from a friend, this was my first time attending. I walked into the studio and saw women and a few men chatting and hugging one another. I signed up for the class, rented a yoga mat, put my personal belongings away, and headed into the room where I was greeted with fifteen students on their mats, some sitting upright and a few in headstand poses. The Russian teacher came in, introduced herself, asked if there were any physical concerns she should be aware of, and then proceeded with the words, "let's start in Child's Pose." Well, being new to yoga, I had no idea of what to do or what the Sanskrit words the Russian yoga teacher was saying meant. What I did know is that the type of yoga I was practicing that morning was nothing like the yoga I had seen on TV and heard about from friends.

For me as a first time yoga student, it was about listening and looking at the other students performing on their mats so I could get a general idea of what to do and how to pose. I was steadfast in my practice and started thinking about when I was a cheerleader in grade school, and of my younger, fluid body. I started thinking how being vegan and not taking nor relying on asthma medications allowed me to push through. Did I mention the room was hot and by the time the hour passed, I had felt amazing? So much so that after the class I signed up for a thirty-day unlimited yoga pass in which I returned every day—except for weekends.

Soon after that, I signed up for a Forty Days to Personal Revolution course. This program was a breakthrough program to radically change my body and awaken the sacred within my soul, with principals founded by Baron Baptiste, founder of Baptiste Yoga. Participating in this course caused me to step out of my comfort zone. I mean, not only was I new to yoga, I also didn't recognize any of the faces—but I quickly connected with like-minded women. The program consisted of practicing yoga every day for forty days, engaging in a three-day guided fruit fest, daily mediation and daily journaling. It was *Ohhmazing* and provided the physical and emotional detox I needed.

By that time, I was hooked on yoga and elevated my yoga practice by registering for yoga teacher training. I was only interested in teacher training to deepen my yoga practice. However, the intensity, spirit, impeccable insight, and knowledge gained from the essence of yoga and a community of fifty-one other yoga students changed my life forever. I was engaged in seven months of yoga, leaving my family while I attended yoga teacher training once a month and spending the entire weekend practicing, studying, and learning all about yoga. It was emotional, grueling, authentic, exhilarating, peaceful, fantastic, and raw. I mean yoga teacher training caused me to drop what I thought I knew and to step out of my comfort zone into something new.

One profound aspect of my yoga teacher training was for me to get clear about who I am, what I represent, and what I want for my life. For me, that meant to become truly authentic, raw-like, and natural. I started yoga teacher training with an entire head full of extensions— or weave. I ended yoga teacher training embracing and wearing my natural hair. It was liberating to say the least. While most may think this was an easy transition, it wasn't for me because I had worn extensions for a very long time. Most black women define themselves by their hair, but I took all of it out after years of having extensions with lengths to the middle of my back. Yoga made me get raw and authentic about who I really am, what I am capable of, and how my actions affect my life. It started in my mind, body, and spirit on the mat, and for that reason, I am forever grateful!

While in teacher training, I met some *Ohhmazing* women who I am still connected to today. I was also offered the opportunity to teach at a local yoga studio while in yoga teacher training. So we are talking about this forty-seven-year-old new yoga student/teacher teaching at a bona fide yoga studio, with lots of students eager to practice on their mats. Me? Yes, me! And I was more than ready and thrilled, scared, and excited. Did I mention yoga caused me to step out of my comfort zone? Not only did I teach yoga at the studio—and found my "voice" while teaching—I was also offered the position to teach yoga for the Canyon Ranch Institute in Tucson, AZ, by way of Savannah, GA.

The privilege of teaching yoga, stress management, mediation, and facilitating to Savannah's inner city public housing/low-income communities was priceless. I am forever grateful to the cause as I support the efforts and work alongside the country's doctor, the 17th US Surgeon General, Dr. Richard Carmona, and president of Canyon Ranch Institute, in an effort to promote health literacy and prevention for people with health disparities. His executive team in partnership with Charles and Rosalie Morris' Connect Savannah, and Albert Grandy, Jr. as CEO of the Curtis V. Cooper Primary Health Care has been relevant and life changing for many.

To me, yoga means unity. Yoga is love. Yoga is peace. Yoga is the ability to share and transform lives through its practices of mediation, asana, and inquiry. Here are the twelve laws of transformation I've incorporated into my life. I hope you take a moment to say these words and then allow these words to connect with your soul:

- seek the truth
- be willing to come apart
- step out of your comfort zone
- commit to growth
- shift your vision
- drop what you know
- relax with what is
- remove the rocks
- don't rush the process
- be true to yourself
- be still and know
- understand that the whole is the goal

These are the principles I learned from practicing, studying, and teaching Baptiste yoga and what I share with my family, friends, students, and clients.

Find time in your busy day to sit in a comfortable position with your legs crossed. Bring your hands to the top of your knees, with thumbs and index fingers to touch. Close your eyes and take three deep breaths. As you breathe in, say the words, "I AM." As you breathe out, say, "YOGA." Take a full breath in and say the words, "I AM," and during your exhalation say, "PEACE." Take a deep breath in and say, "I AM." Breathe all the way out and say the word, "LOVE." Open your eyes slowly as you say the words, "I AM YOGA." Namaste.

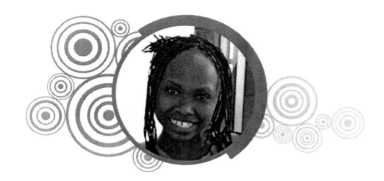

Catherine Njeri, AYP, CBYT

I am a certified Africa Yoga Project (AYP) teacher and a certified Baptiste yoga teacher. I have been teaching Baptiste power vinyasa yoga since 2009. I have done Level 1, 2, and 3 yoga teacher trainings with Baron Baptiste. I am the director of teachers at AYP and a proud mother.

CHAPTER 5

EMBRACING THE CHANGE

By Catherine Njeri, AYP, CBYT

There are many benefits of practicing yoga. The combination of breath and movement leaves one relaxed and flexible, not only in their physical body but also in their mind. Yoga is a practice that is in the body, and I bring yoga everywhere I go.

For people who are on the move most of the time, yoga can be used as a tool to ground their bodies and minds. I took my first yoga class in 2007, and when I got to the class I had no idea what yoga was, as I'd never even heard of the word *yoga*. Something in that class about being strong in myself and in my body showed me that I had the power to change myself. That day was the turning point in my life. I started substituting my acrobatic warm-ups with yoga and two years later, I was in yoga teacher training boot camp!

I grew up in Kariobangi, next to the Korogocho slum, which is the second biggest slum in East Africa. I was raised by a single mum who, by the time I was a teenager, was an alcoholic. My mum lost her job and being the first born, I was left to provide for my family of five at the age of fifteen years. I was still in school and jobless, so I made money by doing other peoples' hair on the weekends and asking for money from the men I pretended to be a girlfriend to, just to put food on the table for my siblings. I hated my mum for being irresponsible and could barely talk to her. After high school, which I was only able to attend because of well-wishers and scholarships, I joined an acrobatic group to keep myself busy, and also to earn a little money. Paige, the founder of Africa Yoga Project, introduced me to Baptiste power yoga, and this practice completely changed my life. I found hope when I felt mostly hopeless.

Africa Yoga Project (AYP) is a nonprofit based in Nairobi, Kenya, and we are changing lives. The organization started in 2009 with a mission of elevating, educating, empowering, and employing youths in Africa. Currently, there are over ninety teachers each teaching five free classes in non-formal settlements in Nairobi.

My relationship with my mum has changed from bad into a great friendship; my mum is now my best friend. Yoga taught me how to let go. I stopped judging and hating my mum for who she was, I accepted what I was going through in my life, and with the help of my friends, my mum changed. She changed because I could understand and she had me to talk to when she was stressed or going through a hard time. My mum is now completely sober and an amazing farmer.

Keeping your body moving in yoga poses is one of the best ways to stay healthy. Getting physically active and sweating at least once a day helps in removing toxins from your body. Yoga is one of the many ways to work out and is my favorite. The best benefits I have received from yoga is self-confidence, understanding, and discipline.

When I was going up in Kenya, the word *compassion* was nowhere to be found. I also had very low self-esteem and was mean to everyone around me. I was full of judgment and I believed what other people said about me. By the time I was leaving the week long yoga teacher training, I was a completely new person and my peers at home noticed the change immediately! Something in the yoga teacher training awakened the true me. I had clarity on what I wanted to do with my life—to work for Africa Yoga Project, the organization that sponsored my teacher training, and to share yoga with my community. I changed my perspective and started seeing things from another angle. I started relating my experience on the mat to my day-to-day life. Poses like Half Pigeon, which is a hip opener, taught me to be patient and to let go of things I could not control—like other people. I am now able to listen to people with positivity and my confidence is great. I am now able to teach a yoga class with three hundred people in the Shine Center—a wellness center created by the Africa Yoga Project—and ask for feedback. When the fear of judgment shows up, I simply remind myself of who I am—a leader! My language has changed from being rude into a compassionate listener.

Africa Yoga Project is giving opportunities to youths like me to be great leaders in their communities. I was shy and didn't care about others. Now I am a leader in my community and my greatest passion in this world is to create leaders. Yoga has given me that opportunity. I lead yoga teacher trainings at AYP and am part of the leadership team in Nairobi. Me being a YES and getting the courage to take that first yoga class has changed my life and the life of my family — two of my sisters are professional yoga instructors now.

Listed above are the benefits of yoga and I am grateful I was open to something new through the practice and teaching of yoga. If I changed and am now changing the world, you can change. Just trust and believe in yourself and the rest will follow.

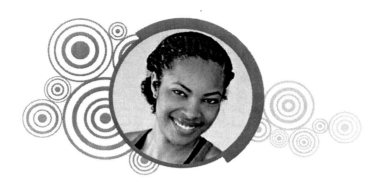

Courtney Waring, RYT

I AM love. Loving yourself is power. I had to learn what love was, the hard way. Who I am and what I do is always done in love with good intentions. Born on Valentine's Day, you could say love is my dharma (life's purpose) and I would have to agree. Without trials and obstacles, there is no story, no testament. I'd like to think all I endured in my childhood had a purpose—to get me here, writing my words of loves' embrace. My dharma is to be a light for love. I AM love. - CourtneyYoga (Waring)

 facebook.com/courtney.yoga.75?fref=ts

 courtneyyoga

CHAPTER 6

YOGA FOR TEENS

By Courtney Waring, RYT

Yoga is a gift. A gift meant to be taught and passed on to future generations. I speak from my own experience—yoga literally saved my life.

Teenage years are filled with confusion and disassociation. Yoga is a journey of the self—through the self, to the self. Learning our true power and who we are as teenagers is the best gift ever!

In my teenage years, I was battling myself more than anything, trying to figure out where I fit in. High school was hell; I would not relive those four years if I was paid to. Due to my upbringing, I did not know what real love or acceptance felt like, so as a result, when someone tried to show me love or acceptance, it was an unfamiliar emotion that I didn't know how to process, let alone handle.

I had abandonment issues. I did not bond with my biological mother when I was born because she handed me off to my grandmother. My grandmother was a beautiful loving soul. She was overweight and disabled. She taught me what love felt like. She taught me how to sew, cook, and love. She did her best by me. When I was with her, she showed me as much love possible considering she had ten other grandchildren in and out of the house. When I hugged my biological mother, there was no feeling there. I felt that warm cozy feeling of love from my grandmother. My biological father is still unknown to this day, so of course there were also daddy issues.

Those weren't my only issues. I had trust issues too. I didn't know who to trust. I went back and forth between my grandmother and my biological mother so much I didn't know who to trust anymore. I knew my grandmother had health issues and she passed away when

I was twelve. My biological mother physically, verbally, and mentally abused me—and still tries to this day. But I'm not a kid anymore and I am stronger. I know now that people respond to you based on how they feel about themselves. Most of the things people say to you actually have nothing to do with you, it is just a projection. I left my biological mother's home at thirteen and briefly moved in with my eighteen-year-old sister. At fourteen, I adopted my new godparents— the best thing that ever happened to me.

As a result of my childhood, I had very low self-esteem. I wondered why I wasn't good enough to be loved by my biologically mother. After all, she gave birth to me. If she didn't love me, then I must not be worthy of love. Maybe I didn't deserve to be loved.

I was holding onto all of baggage—the pain of years of abuse, abandonment, and neglect. It caused me to have major health problems when I was twenty years old. I was on a lot of medication— antidepressants, sleep aids, pain and anxiety medication, and more.

As teenagers, we suffer in silence. We don't think anyone will understand. Not everyone has the same struggles, but as a teen, when you're being introduced to your emotions, it can seem like the world is stacked up against you.

Teaching yoga to teenagers has been a blessing to me. I give them the tips that I wish an adult would have given me. We don't get a handbook, but hints and tips along the way are *gold*. We all need mentors. I still have mentors and will always have mentors. We don't have to burn ourselves to know that the fire is hot—there is someone else that has already burned themselves.

Yoga is a discovery of who you really are. It's a means to an end. Once you learn who you are, no one and nothing can stop you but you. It's a challenge. Life's not easy, but neither is yoga. It's a mental training ground to prepare you for the world.

The most important lesson I have learned from yoga so far is how to hear and trust my gut instinct, because our gut instinct is our steering wheel. It's our guiding force that will lead us to limitless heights and push us to realize our potential. That gut feeling we get when we know that our actions are wrong is the God inside, poking us. We usually talk ourselves through it and make it seem right to us in our own little world. Thing is, we are not in our own little world—we are in one large world where one thing affects the other, and trusting our gut sets up a domino effect of things to come. During an hour of yoga, you get a glimpse of how you think. Our thoughts are influenced by the outside world, and our perspective is shaped by our experiences and interactions with other human beings. How we see ourselves and perceive ourselves comes from how others see and perceive us.

Yoga teaches us to quiet our thoughts and listen to our gut instinct— the God inside. Your first thought is always the right thought. Yoga teaches you not to second guess yourself or our creator that is guiding us. You learn that you are a seed of the most high creator. Our body is our temple and the spirit of God resides inside all of us. Just like we take on characteristics of our mothers and fathers, we take on characteristics of our creator. We are creative beings and our power is limitless when we have good intentions. What we think sends out a vibrational frequency that creates our reality and contributes to the universe as a whole. What you think is what you believe. Do you go to positive or negative thoughts when things get challenging? How do you talk to yourself when you perceive something as being complicated? Self-talk is important because that's where you create the person you are.

I am is the most powerful statement you can make to yourself. Define yourself *for yourself* every morning before you start your journey into this world—as a declaration and reminder of who you are. I am Powerful. I am Love. I can do anything. I fear nothing. I am! We are amazing beings made in the image of our creator, and powerful beyond measure. We must remind ourselves daily of whom we are because it is easy to forget when going through the trials and obstacles of this world. Start by seeing all of your sorrows, trials, and upsets as obstacles. Like an obstacle course, strengthening your faith in yourself and God. Each obstacle we successfully pass makes us stronger physically, mentally, and spiritually. My faith grows leaps and bounds because I am reminded that the creator brought me through yet again. I stay focused on where the ultimate decisions come from—my God, my Creator, my Mother and Father in Heaven, the Universe. Yoga is a tool to constantly remind yourself.

Once you began your journey into yourself through yoga, you began to understand the importance of a strong foundation. You get a stronger understanding of who you are and the power of who created you. In yoga, you push yourself to your edge and then go past your edge and create a new you. That's the foundation of who we are. We never stop growing, we never stop learning. The only thing that matters is this moment here. What you are doing in this moment is defining who you are and how you think for the remainder of your existence. We have an opportunity in every moment of every day to strengthen our foundations. Who said foundations can't be reinforced on an already-built structure? Our foundations are built on the knowing that we are God seeds. We have the biggest and strongest creator in the universe, literally. Just like you will protect your own creations, our creator will always protect us.

Learning to focus and channeling your energy comes from yoga. Your thoughts are energy waves. What you think of most is what you are creating. Channel your energy and set your focus on all things positive. Fill your life with positive thoughts and actions that make you smile and bring your heart joy. Set your focus on what you want to accomplish, keep your eyes set on the prize, and understand that anything else that comes up is just another obstacle to make you stronger.

I started practicing yoga as a way to get off all of my medication. At the time, I thought it was just a physical practice, but after my first class, I learned that it is far more. It's a healing practice. It healed all of the pain I was carrying around. It healed my mind and how I thought about myself, life, and God. As a result of healing my mind, I felt the physical results of my body healing as well. I've never felt better and I practice three times a week. It's my time, to channel my thoughts and focus on healing ME. Channeling your thoughts with loving energy makes them manifest faster. *Quantum physics*, the *law of attraction*, and *karma* are all different terms describing the same ancient concept: WE CREATE OUR REALITY. I learned this and more from yoga. I am a stronger human being because of my practice, and I take this to teens because it makes them stronger adults.

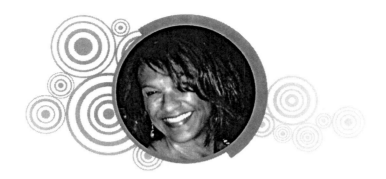

Jacqui Jackson-Young,
RN, BSN, MA, CNWB, HE

Jacqui has worked to help others learn to "take charge" of their health. As a registered professional nurse, she has worked in various specialties both on the front line in acute health care settings, as well as in administrative, educational, and entrepreneurial roles. Jacqui and husband Ronald founded an adult day center and case management company in the Hilton Head, SC, area after semi-retirement from SUNY Upstate Medical University, NY. She is a certified white belt Nia practitioner who has brought Nia to various settings that support the mental, spiritual, and physical health of seniors. Jacqui is an accomplished health instructor and speaker, holding clinical certifications and having had life experiences that have indelibly formed her interest as a wellness enthusiast. A graduate of Syracuse University's College of Nursing, Jacqui has integrated her life experiences and educational expertise to become a well-rounded health care professional, now living in Southern California.

CHAPTER 7

LISTEN TO YOUR BODY. TRUST YOUR BODY. TAKE CHARGE OF YOUR HEALTH

By Jacqui Jackson-Young, RN, BSN, MA, CNWB, HE

When thinking about health and wellness and my "message," I consistently return to my guiding mantra, that which leads me through the worst and best of times in this life journey: "Keep moving forward and do what it is that makes you happy."

As a young girl, my parents must have seen that kinetic energy within me that may have driven them a little crazy! As such, I had to practice the piano daily and take ballet lessons. Their commitment to having their only child be "cultured" probably set a great foundation. I can recall that when my piano teacher selected songs for me to learn and play, I would obediently practice them for the obligatory half hour. But boy oh boy, after that, the improvisation began! I would hum and sing and shimmy all over that piano bench to the Beatles, Rolling Stones, Supremes, and Temptations.

On Saturday mornings, ballet was the obligation and somehow, my soul just didn't sing. As such, I didn't fly, create, or glow. Little did I know that my mind, body, and spirit connection was not being fulfilled between eight and twelve years old. The movement was prescribed and didn't speak to my small body at the time. I would watch the professional ballerinas and wonder how and why they found joy in their art.

During my formal and experiential/life education, the question of holistic health and healing resonated with me. As friends and family passed away or transitioned in other ways, I struggled with how we all merge our spiritual, emotional, and physical health and how intrinsically interwoven these aspects of our lives must be. Without a balance between any three, the homeostasis that we need cannot be achieved. The dictionary defines *homeostasis* as: "the tendency of a system, especially the physiological system of higher animals, to maintain internal stability, owing to the coordinated response of its parts to any situation or stimulus that would tend to disturb its normal condition or function." My translation: *balance*.

We all seek that balance so that our "normal condition or function" may be maintained. We may seek that balance in unhealthy ways, knowingly or unwittingly. We may adapt to situations by eating in unhealthy ways, drinking too much, not exercising, or even taking drugs to stimulate or minimize our emotional or physical reactions to life and its' many changes. Our bodies will respond in ways that let us know that we have not been kind to it and we are not in balance.

I submit to you that you listen to your body, trust that your body will let you know when it is out of balance, and take charge of your own health.

I was introduced to a wonderful practice called Nia in early 2005, while working in an administrative role at a teaching hospital in Upstate New York. When I was encouraged to attend my first Nia class, I kept asking what this was "Nia thing" was all about. My friend kept replying that I needed to "just come and check it out; words can't describe this type of exercise." To best explain Nia, I would direct you to the "Nianow" website (www.NiaNow.com). There you will find this following explanation of Nia and be able to witness demonstrations and read testimonials.

WHAT IS NIA?

"Nia is a sensory-based movement practice that draws from martial arts, dance arts and healing arts. It empowers people of all shapes and sizes by connecting the body, mind, emotions and spirit. Classes are taken barefoot to soul-stirring music in more than 48 countries. Trainings teach people how to workout without pain and enjoy the process of getting fit with movement. Every experience can be adapted to individual needs and abilities.

THE NIA EXPERIENCE

The Nia experience is how we describe the sensation of taking a Nia class. Typically Nia classes include 55 minutes of movement to diverse music.

Nia dance cardio fitness classes are taught by instructors licensed in the Nia Technique. Each class includes mindful movement guidance and somatic education; class cycles include warm-up, sustained non-impact aerobic conditioning, strength training, cool down and stretching. Nia Fitness classes are taught to music, including pop, electronica, jazz, Latin, New Age, Indian and hip hop. They employ 52 basic movements and techniques that draw on a combination of Jazz, Modern and Duncan Dance styles, Tai Chi, Tae Kwon Do and Aikido; and the body-mind healing arts of Feldenkrais Method, Alexander Technique and Yoga." (https://nianow. com/practice, 2014)

I joyfully continued to practice and enjoy life with Nia in 2005 and 2006. The little girl that practiced at the piano for hours and tried to throw her legs onto that ballet bar had found her niche, some forty-plus years later! The joy of movement (our first white belt principle in Nia) filled my soul. To go to a Nia class, you experience the gamut of emotions while increasing your body's strength and awareness. Increasing power, control, and balance and finally reaching a sense of peace occurred in each Nia class I attended.

In late 2006, I noted a nagging pain under my left armpit. As an RN, I knew the possibilities of what this may be. However, having had mammograms every year due to my fibrocystic disease, I trusted that any breast cancer possibility did not exist and if it did, would be diagnosed quickly. My body—and oldest daughter—continued tell me to get further diagnostic testing. When diagnosed with Stage III breast cancer, which had metastasized to several lymph nodes, we were all shocked. I had not eaten beef or pork in twenty-five years, had purposely lost twenty pounds, weighing in at 128, and exercised regularly through my Nia practice—yet my body had let me down! Or had it really? I believe my lymph nodes were keenly capturing those cancerous cells that were attempting to move to other organs.

The ache in my armpit was my "call to arms." Surgery, chemotherapy, and radiation treatments continued throughout 2007, fighting the dreaded triple-negative type of breast cancer.

My wonderful husband, daughters, and friends supported me throughout our battle with the big "c"—and no, that's not a typo! I refuse to capitalize that "c" in this context. Amazingly, my Nia community was one of the lifelines that I held onto throughout the journey. Every Saturday morning, I would get up (sometimes the day after chemo), put on my Nia gear, and travel to my local Nia class. Ellen, my wonderful Nia teacher, greeted me with her knowing smile and continued the class. I tried wearing a bandana to cover my bald head—however, the movement and sweat won that battle of aesthetics. I pulled the scarf off, threw my head back, and continued to dance and soar with the freedom that my spirit needed. No wigs or pieces of cloth to bind or hide the fact that I was healing holistically after Western medicine had provided the chemo and radiation to jump start the healing process.

When practicing Nia, it is important to not let your brain get in the way; the body needs to learn its own parameters and needs and will respond intuitively to what movement is required at the time. Before cancer, I was able to take my Nia moves to a deep level of balance and movement. After surgery, chemo, and radiation treatments, my body ached and many of the nerves in my feet and hands were compromised and numbed due to neuropathy. As such, at first, I was not able to move as deeply and effectively as I wanted. Seven years later, I still find that I do not have the crispness and balance that I was used to. But, guess what?! The beauty of Nia is that there is not "right" or "wrong" way to move! It's your body's way, based on whatever level of ability of stamina that you have at the moment. It is structured in some ways, but Nia provides for freedom of expression. The common understanding in your Nia community is that there are no judgments about the way another person is moving. In fact, if you get caught up in looking for the perfect step or move in Nia, you may miss the experience! Those that get it "right" are those in touch with enjoying the movement of the body.

From the piano bench, ballet bar, dance floors, CAT scans, hospital units, and outdoor trails to my barefoot Nia practice studios, I know that Nia makes me happy! I hope that you experience the joy of movement. Keep moving forward, no matter what!

While pursuing my education to become a registered professional nurse, a voice inside my heart, body, and soul kept saying "health is so much more than the science and practice that I am learning!" Maturity and life stepped in and here I am—wiser, healthier, and sharing my experiences! This knowledge base combined with life well lived forms the foundation for my personal and professional practice and inspires me to constantly work on myself and with others to "take charge of your health!"

Chef Lynne Foster

Lynne C. Foster is the corporate R&D chef for Vegetable Juices, Inc., located in Bedford Park, IL. Chef Lynne is VJI's culinary face to the world. In 2001, Chef Lynne launched a consulting company, Lynne Foster, Inc. In addition to running her consulting company, Chef Lynne also led the prepared foods team department of Whole Foods Market from 2005 to 2006, and served as the corporate executive chef for the Culinary Center for Excellence for ConAgra Foods in 2003. She holds an AOS from The Culinary Institute of America and a BBA in business management from University of Massachusetts at Amherst.

CHAPTER 8

I LOVE FOOD

By Chef Lynne Foster

I love to grow it, cook it, and of course, I love to eat food. I am passionate about food and I respect food—always in moderation, to sustain a healthy life and body.

I grew up as an only child but my parents were both from large families. There were aunts, uncles, and cousins in our home on a regular basis. My parents both loved to entertain and passed the tradition on to me. The holidays were always special, and since we lived close to the Jersey Shore, my dad was an avid fisherman and fish was a staple in my home. The turkey at Thanksgiving was always accompanied by a large blue fish stuffed with crab and shrimp. At Christmas, mussels marinara and baked mackerel with buttered lime sauce were my dad's favorites. He used to say, "Swam in the ocean last night, swim in my stomach tonight!"

Family and friends would gather at our home during the holidays, sharing their favorite dishes to embellish the main course—Aunt Clara's chicken and dumplings, John's ox tail soup, Granny Della's banana pudding, and Uncle Chick's beer battered fish were some of my beloved favorites that bring back fond memories.

It was natural to pursue a career in food to maintain the feelings of joy and satisfaction I get when preparing food and seeing the pleasure it brings to others.

I look at food in stages—growing, cooking, and eating. I'll start with growing and how to flavor.

Every year, I have friends and family who ask about herbs—how to use them, when to plant, and how to pair with food. Well, these are my personal favorites. I hope you too have your own favorite list.

Growing: The following is a list of herbs I plant wherever we live. I use them just like salt and pepper. Refer to your zone guide for proper planting guidelines based on the state you live in. My husband Joel's job has moved us from NJ, AZ, NE, and NY. Now we reside in IL. So knowing when to plant outside is important. You can also plant indoors as long as there is enough sunlight. However, I prefer outdoors so the plants can reach their maximum potential growth.

Plants are either annuals—which must be planted every year, or perennials—which return every year on their own.

Basil (annual) – The Italian finishing herb. Put on almost any Italian dish once it's finished cooking, such as bruschetta (which is really what the bread is called but we refer to the chopped tomatoes, olive oil, garlic, and balsamic). Great for: salads, pasta, pesto. Try Thai basil for anything Thai.

Cilantro (annual) – The Mexican herb. Good on salsa. Prepared the same as bruschetta, except cilantro instead of basil, and lime instead of balsamic. Great for: Pico de gallo, black bean soup, rice, chicken, and fish.

Sage (perennial) – The cooking herb. Great for: chicken, butternut squash, or most winter squash. If you plant this, it makes beautiful lavender blooms.

Rosemary (annual) – The meat and root vegetable herb. Great for: chicken, lamb, carrots, beets, and sweet potatoes.

Dill – (annual or perennial, depending on location) - The pickle herb. Great for: cucumbers and salmon.

Parsley (annual) – The king of finishing herbs. Put it on everything. Great for: the digestive system.

Thyme (perennial) – The Cajun herb. Great for: chicken, meat, potatoes, and most root vegetables.

Oregano (perennial) – The Italian herb. Great for: anything Italian, then finish with parsley. When planting outside, be careful, as it returns every year larger than the previous year. Don't be afraid to trim back because it can take over a garden.

Tarragon (perennial) – The delicate herb. Great for: Fish, chicken, and in creamy salad dressings. I love it in my tuna salad.

Lavender (annual) – The lovely herb. I just love to smell it. Great for: custards. Or just boil on the stove to make the house smell good. Place in sachet bag with Epsom salt and put in your bath. You can even wash your floors with it, really!

My favorite vegetables to plant: tomatoes, cucumbers, lettuce (romaine, Bibb, butter) assorted peppers, green beans, and collards. Always try a new vegetable in the garden. Here are a few: watermelon (keep elevated), pumpkin (watch out for squirrels, they love it!), sweet potatoes, onions, and beets (ask your local greenhouse when to harvest since these are root vegetables and the leaves are so beautiful you'll be tempted to leave them in the ground too long—at least I was!).

Planting vegetables and maintaining a garden brings a sense of peace. I don't listen to my iPod, or talk on my phone because it's quiet time to connect with the earth and be in touch with God and nature. Turning off technology and caring for the garden is so calming and Zen-like; I know exactly what's going on with my plants—who is thriving, who looks a little sad, and who is being bothered by pests. I believe in organic soil and natural pesticides. When you care for a garden in this way, the harvest will always be plentiful and the labors few. There is always work to do maintaining a healthy garden, so think of it as a natural workout!

Cooking: There aren't enough words to describe my feelings. Peace, love, and therapy are a few that come to mind. The balancing and layering of flavors that excite our taste receptors is a craft that can be learned by consistently experimenting with cooking all types of food. Sweet, salty, sour, and savory notes can work in complete harmony, like a symphony orchestra playing a wonderful piece of music— strings, woodwinds, brass, and percussions. For example, a simple dish like soup has basic ingredients: vegetables, broth, protein, and seasoning. The strings are the high notes forming the basis of the music, much like the vegetables that are used when starting a soup. The woodwinds support the high notes, carrying the melody, much like broth that is added to vegetables. The brass section also supports with tempo, enhancing the soup by seasoning with herbs and spices. And finally, there are the percussions, which carry the beat and form the background—the overall savory character from the meat or protein. I am the conductor, helping the ingredients play together, getting the right balance so that the soup can be fully enjoyed.

Eating: Food is essential for life and should be fully enjoyed. However, we should also have respect for food and our bodies. Being fully cognizant of the food we eat and how much we eat is something we shouldn't take for granted. There are so many that don't have the privilege of having enough food or enjoying their food. This is why I am so grateful and thankful to enjoy food and work in the food industry. After growing and cooking, eating our creations is the best part—it gives us energy and satisfies our hunger. It should also be a time to think about keeping our bodies healthy by eating nutritious food. Of course, there are times when we want to indulge on fatty foods or sweets, like ice cream, but we should keep those to a minimum and try to increase the fruits, vegetables, and complex carbohydrates in our diets. Many of the recipes I will share focus on vegetables and whole grains, which I combine with sweet and savory sauces.

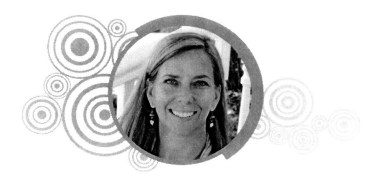

Tisha Chafer, CHHC

Tisha Chafer is a full time Sales Consultant for David Weekley Homes, a mother of two busy beautiful teenagers, two dogs, and one guinea pig. She is married to a handsome Australian she picked up 20 years ago in Ohio, whose hobby is Ironman Triathalon. When not working or watching her children play competitive sports Tisha works on her health coaching business through her blog and websites. She is a graduate of Ohio University earning a BSC in Communications in 1992, and The Institute for Integrative Nutrition, receiving her certification as a Holistic Health Coach in 2014. Tisha Resides in Bluffton, South Carolina and enjoys yoga, tennis, running, gardening, green smoothies and all things related to health and wellness.

www.tishwellness.com

www.GSGlife.com

✉ tishwellness101@gmail.com

f Green Smoothie Gal

🐦 @tishachafer

CHAPTER 9

TIPS FOR THE BUSY WORKING MOM
By Tisha Chafer, CHHC

Being a mother is not easy—whether you are a stay-at-home mamma bear or a corporate tiger juggling kids and boardroom drama. It's hard work. Hectic, frazzled moms on the run in our society are considered a normal site. I'm not talking about running from the police here either (although the rebel side of me yearns for a Thelma and Louise road trip, I won't lie!). I'm talking about our daily schedules. Many of us continuously move from one task to the next from the time we lift our pretty heads off the pillow to the time we finally crumble back into bed in a heap of exhaustion. For working mothers, we have to split our time between taking care of the family and performing at work while trying to do both jobs equally well. It can be a constant struggle with priorities often leaving us feeling spent and depleted, thinking we are not doing either job well. Throw into the mix a desire to eat healthy meals, work out, and embrace sustainable living, and that crunches our time even more.

If you are a busy working mom who is passionate about health and wellness, but find yourself wanting to throw your computer against the wall when you see another Pinterest or Facebook post on a beautifully prepared organic meal by some equally beautiful glowing woman who tells you that "you can do this too"—keep reading. You and I know it's just not as EASY as they make it look, especially when you work eight hours a day outside the home! I love those beautiful, glowing bloggers, but they get my famous eye roll A LOT from me. Who are these women and are they really living in my busy working-mother world?

Their posts about their perfect GMO-free, gluten-free, vegan organic meals that the entire family loves, and how—with just a little bit of organization and farmers-market navigation skill—I can serve this up every night too is one of those things that actually makes me go, "Hmmm." If you are the same, but never wanted to admit it, then you are a part of my tribe and we will be good friends.

Clearly, I'm either too selfish, too unorganized, or too time-crunched to live in this world of BPA-free containers, 100 percent organic living, and home-cooked meals. I've accepted that I really cannot do it all, and I've decided in order to maintain my own health and sanity, I'm not spending my days off in the kitchen meal-prepping for the week. I told you I was selfish, but I'm perfectly OK with that. I know I'm much more loving, caring, and a better person when I take the time to participate in the activities that I enjoy. Keep me from the tennis courts, the gym, yoga, my writing, or a road trip for too long and I'm not someone you want to have around.

So, do we continue to sacrifice the wellness of ourselves and families because we feel it's too difficult to live up to all of this healthy living? If we can't be "all in" and do it all perfectly, why try at all?

I say absolutely not to sacrificing the wellness of ourselves and our families! We know that food is medicine. Our bodies need and crave the right nourishment and exercise, and our minds need peace, stillness, and quiet. I say we do not have to resign ourselves to feeling inadequate when we cannot live up to the expectations that we are really imposing on ourselves. Those nice holistic bloggers are only trying to be light and love to us. They don't judge us—we judge ourselves!

Our kids do not have to be raised on processed junk food or be strung out on red dye and rivers of soda. Working moms do not have to give in to the grab-and-go fast food mentality that wreaks havoc on our bodies. We can allow ourselves to be selfish *and* practice self-care and not feel ONE BIT GUILTY about it.

These are things I have realized while working full-time and trying to embrace a healthier lifestyle. I don't do it all perfectly, but I've learned to be diligent about the things I *can do* at this season in my life—and not waver from them.

My top three "easy and healthy habits for women on the go" are easy to incorporate into your everyday busy lives. I know, it sounds like another one of those blog posts—but I promise you, it's not. I like to tell clients to start small and build upon each step. Or, pick one and stick with it! What I have learned is that when you choose to do something, and you remain disciplined about that practice, the results do come. Health does come, weight loss does come, a clearer focused mind does come, and a refreshed version of yourself emerges. Beauty can and will rise from the ashes. I promise.

OK, so here we go for three easy steps for the busy working mom and her family...

Step 1: Hop on the green smoothie train. Why? Because greens are filled with good stuff our bodies need—like chlorophyll, magnesium, folic acid, and tons of vitamins and minerals. Look at gorillas; they eat pounds of leafy greens every day and they are strong, intelligent, and lean creatures. No one wants to mess with a gorilla, right? They are not eating pizza, beer, wine, fast food, and cereal. Greens...they eat greens!

My favorite part about green smoothies for busy moms is that they are fast and easy to make. All you need is a blender and some fruit and veggies. Once you get the hang of it, you can then start adding cool "super-food" items like chia seeds, spirulina, maca powder, and goji berries. You can whip up a smoothie, drink it in the carpool line, and freak out all the kids with the bright green stuff you're guzzling.

Here is my favorite green smoothie recipe:

1/2 cup of filtered water
1 cup of pineapple
1 cup of mango
Heaping handful of spinach and kale, or just spinach
1/2 cup of fresh cilantro
1/2 inch of fresh ginger

Fresh fruit is always best, but I don't have time in the morning to deal with a fresh mango, so we use frozen—and we are still alive and kicking.

Step 2: Eat like a gorilla. Why? See above. Do you want to be a lean, mean, woman machine? Maybe, maybe not, but what could be easier to throw together for your own lunch to take to work than some greens with tons of veggies on it? Ditch the frozen meals, please—they are not good for you—and stock your refrigerator with spinach, kale, arugula, romaine, and fresh veggies every week and make yourself EAT them! If you are like me and would rather drink your food than eat it, blend it all up again and take another smoothie, or make a pot of veggie soup and put it in those BPA-free containers you have stocked up on. Benefits? Besides being filled with cancer-fighting carotenoids, flavonoids, iron, vitamin K, calcium, and other healthy things I can't pronounce, I love them because they really help to curve my cravings for sweets. For a 1-2 punch against that sweet tooth, add sweet veggies to your green leafy salad. Try beets, roasted butternut squash, roasted pumpkin, and fresh avocado. Load up on all this goodness and watch that sweet tooth slowly disappear.

Step 3: Stock up with healthy quick-cooking essentials. This has been key for me. I know if I have the essentials in my pantry and fridge, I can whip up a healthy meal in no time for the family, even if I get home late. My ten basic items are:

1. Quinoa: It takes fifteen minutes to cook and is very versatile—add spices and veggies for flavor.

2. Brown rice: Invest in a rice cooker. It's the best investment ever for the kitchen (besides a fancy blender).

3. Black beans: You can do anything with these things—burgers, salsa variations, throw them on salads, and more...

4. Sodium-free canned tomatoes: Great for quick pasta dishes and soups.

5. Rice noodles: Perfect to combine with diced veggies for quick stir fry

6. Plant-based protein powder: When I don't feel like cooking, it's protein shakes for dinner.

7. Organic ground meat or range free chicken: I'm not a vegan or vegetarian and that is OK.

8. Free-range eggs: I'm famous for "breakfast for dinner" (when making pancakes, I use buckwheat pancake mix).

9. Organic salsa: Combine with grass-fed ground meat and you have meatloaf in fifteen minutes!

10. Frozen veggies: Easier for quick meals, like when you are cooking after sports practices.

As working moms, we are pulled in different directions every day, with little time left to focus on health and wellness. But with just a little thought, effort, and planning, we can be the force of change in our homes. By starting out with these three easy steps, you will be well on your way to feeling great, feeling good about what you are putting into your families bodies, and confident that you are sowing the seeds of a healthy lifestyle mindset for generations to come.

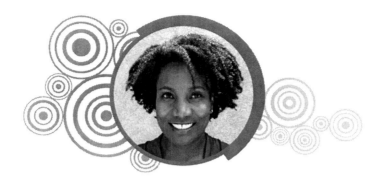

Kenita P. Hill,
MSA, CPHRM, LNHA, LPN

Kenita is a devoted wife and proud mother of three boys. She has a master's degree in health services administration from Central Michigan University and a BS in health planning and management and business administration from Alfred University. Kenita is a certified professional healthcare risk manager, a licensed nursing home administrator, and an LPN. As a caregiver for the elderly, Kenita has seen firsthand the negative power of choosing to hold onto baggage and the detrimental impact it can have on one's life. Her intention in participating in this incredible project is to encourage women to let go of past hurts and live a happy, fulfilled life.

CHAPTER 10

LET IT GO AND LIVE

By Kenita P. Hill, MSA, CPHRM, LNHA, LPN

"When you hold on to your history, you do it
at the expense of your destiny."

~ T.D. Jakes

A dear friend and I were having lunch and discussing the amount of people we know who were dealing with emotional pain from past relationships—painful experiences that resulted from co-workers who talked behind their backs; family members who cast unwarranted judgments; and spousal betrayals. What was interesting is how they chose to handle their situations. Many had their bad experience years ago and you would have thought the incident occurred yesterday because their wounds were still so fresh. They remembered the day, time, and every detail of those traumatic, life-changing moments. Others walked away from their experiences wiser, emotionally stronger, and ready to embrace the gifts that life has to offer.

For most women, betrayal from a trusted confidante is a life-changing event. Unfortunately, for many of us, we remain frozen in time… unable to breathe and unable to move. The daily blessings of life are happening all around, yet we can't respond because our world has just fallen apart. Emotions have taken over and rational thoughts are an unattainable concept. We're in a black hole alone with the raw emotions of rage, anger, and hurt. Our soul cries out for something or someone to heal the pain.

Initially, you feel alone, lost, and out of control. Slowly, your world stops spinning and you're finally able to breathe and respond to life around you. Now you have a choice to make: stay lost in the black hole with your emotions, or acknowledge what has happened, take away the lesson to be learned, and move forward to live your life with passion and purpose. Let's examine both options: Living in the black hole versus living a life of peace and purpose.

OPTION 1: LIFE IN THE BLACK HOLE

If you choose to stay immobilized and frozen in the past, you will be comforted by your raw emotions. It is in this cold, barren place where you will grieve over your hurt and harden your heart towards those who have betrayed you. Every detail of those moments will be replayed in your mind, several times a day without fail, guaranteeing your wounds will not heal.

Time will pass but you will be standing still, holding on to past hurts and memories. You have no future because you can only focus on the past. Opportunities for happiness and new experiences present themselves, but you can't see them because they are hidden behind the fog of deception, self-pity, and resentment. It is not possible to attract positive, fulfilling experiences when you're sending out negative energy. No one is attracted to a sad, bitter person who spends their waking hours complaining. We all know someone who people tend to avoid because they sap our energy with their negative attitude.

Your family and friends mourn the loss of the loving and trusting person that you used to be. As you withdraw from them, and into your world of self-pity and sorrow, you close the door to fulfilling relationships and opportunities with your loved ones. They too will withdraw because you are emotionally unstable and they are afraid that the wrong words or gestures will send you plummeting into an emotional crisis.

Don't make the mistake that your children are immune to the effects of your negative energy. They are quickly sucked into your black hole that is void of sincere happiness. No matter how good you think you are, children are very receptive to your energy. A house full of tension is stressful for everyone. The black hole prevents you from sincerely giving and receiving love.

OPTION 2: LET IT GO AND LIVE

If you choose to let go of the past and walk in the present, you understand that you will never reach your destination by looking in the rearview mirror. It's OK to grieve and acknowledge the hurt and anger. You're human. You know that there are lessons to be learned from all of your experiences—good and bad—that strengthens and equips you for life's journey. In addition, you know that living a life of self-pity will guarantee you a life of unhappiness.

Begin your healing process by starting the day being thankful for something, *anything*. Here's a start:

- Being alive
- First sip of coffee in the morning
- The love of family
- Friendships
- The dog or cat that loves you unconditionally
- The sound of laughter
- Your health

Next, live in the moment. So much time is spent on multi-tasking that we miss all of the little blessings that are showered on us every day. Put down your smartphone, step away from your social media of choice, look your loved ones in their eyes when they are talking to you, and enjoy the moment. Take a walk and listen to the birds sing. Life is precious; stop to enjoy it because you will never have this moment again.

Surround yourself with positive people. Spend time with others who are supportive and will encourage you to soar among the eagles. You will never get to higher ground by hanging with the chickens. In addition, take the negative energy off of yourself by doing something positive for others.

Finally, get to know yourself and be at peace with who you are. Know what the triggers are that lead you to the black hole and avoid them. In the event that you can't avoid the trigger, learn how to deal with it and move forward. Don't allow yourself to get sucked into the black hole. Every day we have a choice on how we respond to life's challenges—choose to move forward and enjoy your personal journey.

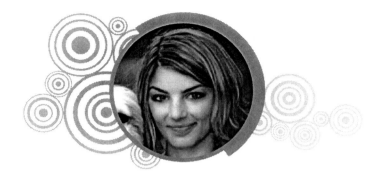

Zoë Zadoorian

Zoë Zadoorian is a senior in high school at Hilton Head Christian Academy. She has a passion for ballet and has been a ballerina for fifteen years. After seeing what girls go through on a daily basis, not only in high school, but in everyday life—including ballet, she decided at the age of seventeen to create Everything Girl, in which she aspires to connect with women ranging from teenagers to the elder women in the community. Zoë relates to these women through her blog, Facebook, and YouTube channel.

everything-girl-beyou.blogspot.com

f **facebook.com/EverythingGirlBEYOU**

▶ **youtube.com/channel/UC1WzOzxCpvjNzztCjxwc3Kg**

CHAPTER 11

THE BOLD STATEMENT IN TEENS

By Zoë Zadoorian

There are many statements that teen girls make in their high school careers, but there is only one they truly care about more than anything in high school. High school is a tough time for us girls because we have so much on our plates. Teen girls are already hormonal, and all they want to do is look pretty. Trust me, I know. I am a high school girl and it is not as fun as everyone says it is. High school is stressful, and all that stress leads to many complications when it comes to beauty in girls' everyday lives. Our skin isn't perfect, our hair is always a mess, and well, our clothes aren't exactly how we want them because "NOTHING SEEMS TO FIT!" So girls and mothers of teen girls, let's take a journey through high school/teen girl beauty…together.

There are moments when you try the cutest clothes on, but "NOTHING SEEMS TO FIT!" You want to scream, cry, and smile all at once, but how can we feel all those things at once…especially about clothes? Well, it's simple really—girls only want the newest, cutest, and most fabulous, high-end fashion out there. So when it doesn't look exactly how it does on Taylor Swift, Selena Gomez, or Miranda Kerr, then we girls just feel lousy about ourselves. I've been through this, and I believe that different stores don't have all the same exact sizes you normally would fit into. If I buy a pair of pants from Victoria's Secret, and then buy the same type of pants from Hollister, the sizes are completely different. Yes, I may wear one size in Victoria's Secret, but in Hollister I may be two sizes bigger. Mothers, we girls are really sensitive about the sizes we wear, so all we want is some reassurance. Girls, don't worry about your size because you are beautiful, and there is no fix to having different sizes. It's just something we will have to live with as girls and as we get older.

Girls, we also have these moments which I like to call "ugly to gorgeous moments," because we feel that our faces look absolutely disgusting, when we probably look gorgeous in our natural form. Sometimes, we apply way too much makeup, which makes our faces look like a mask, and people can't see the true beauty that we cover with over-the-top makeup. High school teens don't need a ton of makeup because yes, we are going through the "pimple face" stage, and when we try to cover up our pimples, which may not even be as bad as we think, it actually makes it worse. Girls, sometimes we just figure out how to use makeup on our own, but we really should be taught how to use the brushes, liners, mascaras, lipsticks, and much more from our mothers—or even YouTube. I don't apply a ton of makeup because I have learned from my mistakes—the less makeup I use, the better I actually look.

So I created my own natural look, which every girl can do. It is very simple. All you have to do is follow these three steps: 1.) Go on YouTube and look for natural looks that resemble your complexion, eye color, and hair color. 2.) DON'T apply foundation all over your face to cover up anything. Use concealer to hide little pimples—but not a lot. 3.) Just find what looks natural on you.

As girls, we can see that it's hard to find a natural look, and we sometimes give up, but with just a little faith in ourselves, and makeup, everything will be fine.

As girls, we hate when our nails don't look perfect, or maybe some of us don't really care what our nails look like. As a young girl, I picked up the ongoing habit of biting my nails, which was probably one of the worst habits I have picked up. I realized that my fingers didn't look like they should. Things just didn't seem to add up. I looked at all of my friends' nails and saw that they had beautiful nails, then I looked at mine and was disgusted. That is the moment I stopped biting my nails because I felt it would be a huge improvement for my girly look, and I felt I was just a lot prettier. I had gel manicures. That actually helped me to make sure I didn't bite my nails, which made everything a little easier. I also had a stress ball that I could hold and it helped, because if I watched a movie that was scary or just dramatic, then I would squeeze my stress ball instead of biting my nails. Also, I came up with the idea of having my phone out, doing something on it—whether it was playing a game or texting my friends, because that actually helped me dramatically. Just keeping my hands busy—with either texting, games, or the stress ball—allowed me to forget about biting my nails. Now, whenever I put my hands close to my mouth, I have no urge to bite them because I love how they look. So girls, if you bite your nails, I promise these methods help with getting rid of that habit.

There is a type of beauty I like to call "the gorgeous heart!" I call it this for a very specific reason. Girls are most beautiful when they have a huge heart and don't bash anyone, for any reason. Girls who have class at a young age, as in being a teenager, are extremely pretty. Wearing short, short skirts and high, high heels and a low-cut top is not classy, but wearing a pencil skirt, heels, and a button-down or collared shirt is very classy,—but that is not the only way girls can have class. The way we present ourselves with our actions and words are what is the classiest part of a girl. A girl who is beyond beautiful can be the nastiest girl out there, and there is no class at all, but a girl who has "the gorgeous heart" will be a much more beautiful girl in the end. The outcomes are different, but class will never go out of style.

The bold statements teens can make are very, very clear to our mothers, and to everyone around us. Being organic in every interaction is what makes a girl beautiful. Makeup, hair, nails, and clothes aren't what makes a girl gorgeous in the long run—it's how she presents herself to others. However, there is no fix to going through all the drama that comes with being a girl, especially when it comes to the beauty side of being a girl. We just have to deal with the growing-up part during high school—being the bigger person no matter what is healthy and beautiful. Yes the outer beauty to high school girls is very important, but what we don't pay attention to is the inner beauty, because we don't think people can hurt us with the inner part of us if we look beautiful on the outside. Except when people do say hurtful things to us, we do get bruised and cut on the inside. The outside may stay strong, but there isn't anything beautiful about people who bruise and cut people on the inside. It just allows girls to lose self-esteem, and losing self-esteem makes us feel even worse about the beauty in our everyday lives. And even though we say we are "fine," sometimes we just aren't fine. Speaking from experience, I can honestly and organically say that high school is just a living hell and we girls just have to suffer through it—but that is why we have our true friends…and class. "The gorgeous heart" isn't just something I made up, it's an honest quality that some girls have, and girls who don't have it can create it because it is what makes us gorgeous. We just have to understand that beauty comes from confidence and loving ourselves unconditionally. Beauty in all aspects comes from the inside, and sometimes it's beautiful if we don't put on a strong outside, and instead, we just show what's going on inside of us. Beauty is something that only we can provide from the self-confidence we have on the inside, and that we portray, not what make-up or anything can do for us. Being organic is beautiful, so let that shine through, and show the true inner beautiful YOU!!!

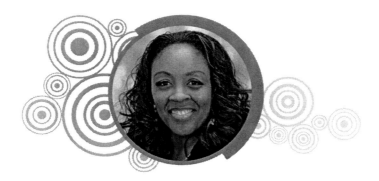

Sheree Darien, CPDC

Sheree Darien—wife, mother, servant enabler, leader, purpose development coach, visionary, excellence provoker, and marketplace minister. Known for her candid delivery and matter-of-fact character, Sheree is a human octopus. With a wealth of life experiences, a plethora of invaluable human relationships and acquired knowledge, Sheree has become a well sought-after center of influence.

This now-entrepreneur, international author, connector of opened doors/opportunities, and radical truth bringer shares her development as a continual process of being broken, molded, and shaped. With childlike-faith, this daddy's girl's mission is to offer others the hope of a second chance.

CHAPTER 12

TOTALLY FREE, TOTALLY ME

By Sheree Darien, CPDC

A prelude into testimony, a second chance. My journey to becoming totally free and totally me! An awakening into the two most important relationships any of us will ever have…

Me: Sitting Indian-style at yet another crossroad, praying to God…

God: Sheree, what do you want? I am not a puppet master. The choice is up to you.

The journey to becoming totally free in my mind, body, and spirit included a state of depression, stress, and a spiritual awakening through a personal relationship with my father. God came that we might have life and live more abundantly. Wholeness is inclusive of being in health, even as our soul prospers...

You see, our journey, simply put, is a process. For me, it seemed like an eternity!

Why? Primarily because I was addicted to my own story. Tears were my way of escape, my safe place, my comfort zone. I was living in crisis management! There was one problem after the other until I got tired of me. And you have to get tired too (if you want to be totally free). Your story does not end here (with hardship, debt, divorce, depression, addiction, etc...). I'm no longer in love with my past. No one wants to die depressed, stressed, and merely existing day by day when God said we can LIVE.

I believe the Bible (all of it). I choose to live by it 24/7. Here is one of my favorite scriptures, which is found in 1 Corinthians 2:9 — "But as it is written, Eye has not seen, nor ear heard, neither have entered into the heart of man, the things which God hath prepared for them that love him." My future looks much better than my past. All of it was necessary and all things are working together for good. My mess is being used as a message to you.

During a leadership trip to Canada four years ago, I was asked a very uncomfortable question. Truthfully, it wasn't the question, but rather my answer to the question. The question was: what type of leader are you? After describing my leadership style, the individual responded, so you are a savior? He went on to say, "But Sheree, don't you know saviors have to be crucified?" I was immediately offended. But it's the truth, and he was right. I saw a glimpse of who I was then.

Total equals wholeness. Second means anything after one. Darling, it is never too late to begin again. However, your freedom is directly connected to a decision. Make one and own it! No regrets; no retreat.

Freedom is liberating. Weights are lifted and removed. When we know better, we are supposed to do better—and we are not supposed to go back to doing those same old things again. Proverbs 26:11 of the Bible compares this type of behavior to a dog returning to its own vomit. Yes, it's disgusting.

We all have a journey, and though each journey is similar, they are all unique to each of us. We are more alike than we are different. It is our uniqueness that makes us special, but it is our likeness that keeps us connected.

Now, it's your turn to give birth. It's time to PUSH through the pain! Pray until something happens...more pain, more power. Luke 12:48 declares, "To whom much is given much is required." It's all about responsibility. Will you abort or will you deliver?

We are all here for a reason. Make YOUR life count. Fill in the blank—the blank space between your birth and your death. Use your unique imprint to make an impact and leave a mark that cannot be erased. Live on purpose. It is time to move from crisis management to purpose management. Your life is 100 percent your responsibility—no one else's. Choose to live, press reset, and recreate your second chance.

Here are a few questions that will hopefully make you uneasy enough to think twice and begin again. Ask yourself: Am I effective or affected? Am I living from one problem to the next? Am I allowing my circumstances to run my life? Am I allowing other peoples' actions to dictate my reaction? Am I expecting others to make me happy? Do I know my purpose? Do I know my worth? Do I know who I am?

Beloved, be willingly to embrace the truth in each answer. Dream!!! Dreams do come true.

Today, I know my worth. I equate my value to the blood Jesus shed on the cross at Calvary. Apart from Him, I am nothing. But in Him, I am inestimable!!! I know that I am loved. I am whole. I am finally free. My mandate is to speak the truth in love, to be transparent, naked, and unashamed.

I am a connector of opportunities and opened doors. My assignment is to have courageous conversations and be OK doing so. I've been crucified, now I must enable others to move into their own second chance (purpose).

My friend, always recognize your motive. Remain pure, honest, and full of compassion. Compassion is defined as a feeling of wanting to help someone who is sick, hungry, in trouble, etc.

You are probably wondering, "How did I make it?" Or possibly saying, "You don't know what I'm dealing with." The only difference is I did not give up. One day, I arrived to a place where epiphany and destiny collided.

Beloved, you must start by changing your confession. I did! I used to say that I had to grow up fast. Now I declare I have an accelerated destiny!!! My good, bad, and ugly story addiction is now my message of hope, encompassing years of innocence, ignorance and deliverance.

Here are a few useful scriptures I live by:

2 Corinthians 1:20 – For all the promises of God in Him are Yes, and in Him AMEN, to the glory of God through us.

Psalm 23:1 – The Lord is my shepherd, I shall not want…

Jeremiah 29:11 – For I know the plans I have for you, declares the Lord, plans to prosper you and not harm you, plans to give you a hope and a future.

Hebrews 13:5 – Let your conduct be without covetousness; be content with such things as you have. For He Himself will never leave you or forsake you.

Proverbs 23:7 – For as he thinks in his heart, so is he...

1 John 4:4 – You, dear children, are from God and have overcome them, because the one who is in you is greater in me than the one who is in the world.

Psalms 56:8 – You keep track of all my sorrows. You have collected all my tears in your bottle. You have recorded each one in your book.

Psalms 30:5 – For His anger is but for a moment, but His favor is for a lifetime or in His favor is life. Weeping may endure for a night, but joy comes in the morning.

Romans 8:18 – Yet what we suffer now is nothing compared to the glory he will reveal to us later.

Your action plan:

- Make a decision!
- Embrace the process and fine tuning.
- Find a Purpose Coach—I'm waiting...
- Be courageous —do not quit! (Feel the pain and do it anyway).
- Use wisdom and expect obstacles.
- Inspect yourself—mirror, mirror—and remove the masks.
- Acknowledge your feelings of intuition. They are your internal compass/radar system.
- Evaluate and shift (your ceiling is becoming your floor—get ready to go to your next level).
- Remain humble—no room for pride or ego!
- Exercise your faith!!!

- Be your own #1 cheerleader. Remember YOU are responsible for YOU.
- Testify!

Revelation 12:11 declares, "We overcome by the blood of the lamb and the word of our testimony."

He even gave me a new name: Sheree bka Kingkid—daughter of the Most High God.

So, who am I? I am emotional, strong-willed, determined, tender-hearted, a servant leader, confident, daddy's girl, classy, transparent, connector, wise, serious, giving, candid, expressive—ALL of the this and yet, I am undone.

I made a decision and I'm still shifting. I purposely choose to be spirit-led and no longer emotionally driven. I am living life on the inside out. On purpose!

You see, in order for me to be totally free and totally me, I first had to decide to be totally accepting of Sheree—all that I am and all that I am not. God sees all of our hind (hidden and private) parts.

Remember, it is according to the power that works in us.

You are SOMEONE SPECIAL, but it's up to you to figure exactly WHO YOU ARE and WHY YOU ARE HERE.

You were BORN alone; you will DIE alone. It's up to you to decide how you will BEGIN to LIVE your life NOW. You can get back on track. It's never too late…seize today!!! Begin again!

Smooches, beloved!!!

I am totally,
Sheree

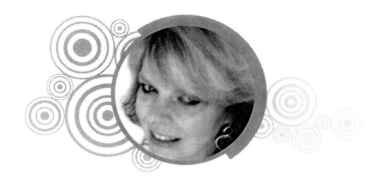

Cathy Shearouse

Born in Petersburg, Virginia, Cathy is a single mother of one daughter, Ansley, a senior at George Mason University. She currently resides in the Hilton Head, SC, area where she is passionately building a career in sales and marketing as local stores marketer for Jim 'N Nick's Restaurants SC Market.

Cathy holds a bachelor of arts degree from Newberry College, where she was named who's who among students in American Universities and Colleges.

Prior to moving to the Hilton Head area, Cathy lived in Tennessee, Virginia, Georgia, and Indiana.

 linkedin.com/pub/catherine-shearouse/43/182/a49

CHAPTER 13

HEALTHY NEW BEGINNINGS

By Cathy Shearouse

Throughout our lives, we ALL will have new beginnings—we may refer to them as new phases, cycles, periods, etc., but all of these phases will ultimately take us to new places in our lives, along with many new relationships. These will be attributed to various life-changing events—empty nest; the death of a close friend, spouse or relative; divorce; major move; career change; etc. In order to transition to this new cycle, it is important that our lives remain in a healthy balance for mind, body, and spirit. For some, this will be easier than for others. I am inspired to share my story with you to hopefully help you transition as you enter a new phase of life and new relationships.

For me, my "new beginning" was due to divorce and was coupled with the loss of three close family members within a seventeen-month period. I will share with you my experiences to teach you about transitioning through these difficult unknown periods and to continue on living life to its fullest—nurturing and developing relationships, and especially, finding out who you are.

Three years ago, I realized that my marriage of twenty-eight years was ending and that I would be starting life over again. My only daughter had just started her freshman year in college at a campus over five hundred miles from our home. The how and why of my marriage ending is not what I wish to share, but what is important is how I was able to move on through this phase of life, becoming an independent single woman and continuing to inspire my daughter day to day to be an independent strong young woman as well. I am writing this to encourage the many of you who are dealing with similar changes in your daily lives. Please know that these changes happen to the "best" of us and that life does GO ON.

First, let me say how important it is as a mother to maintain a close relationship with your children as you transition to new beginnings. You will be comforting and inspiring to each other, sharing your day-to-day activities, trials, and tribulations. My daughter and I are very close. We talk and text almost every day. Although there is quite the difference in age, we now share a very similar parallel in our lives. We are both single women! I have to say, I always thought I would have discussions with my daughter about being a great wife and partner in marriage and relationships as she reached adulthood. However, I did not prepare for discussions about our dates, boyfriends, and fashion for single women. Let me say that my daughter continues to be my strongest inspiration and cheerleader for the single world as we talk, laugh, and share stories about the opposite sex and our daily encounters. Let this be an opportunity to draw closer to your children and to be inspired by their energy, youth, and wisdom.

One of the biggest positive changes in my life over the past three years is that I began a daily workout with a personal trainer. Incorporating a daily workout in your life and following a healthy balanced diet is extremely important. Having a personal trainer and daily cardio workout has been one of the best changes I have made in my life. It has truly contributed to making me a better person, mentally and physically, through the transition and has helped me deal with the challenging, difficult days. It is great to have a focus of personal goals for both your health and appearance. I have also developed relationships and connected with many people who also share the same goals.

I have learned to embrace family and close friends. It is OK to allow yourself to share a part of your life with those that are close to you. In doing this, please know you will be given a lot of advice and coaching. Learn to be grateful for these gifts and take the advice needed for you and move on. Remember that everyone gives advice from their own personal experience and knowledge. This will come in different shapes and sizes from each person.

One of the most eye-opening things I've learned as a single woman is that there are now "cheerleaders" in my life, and how vital it is to accept these people in my life, allowing their words and comments to inspire me daily. Open your heart and mind to sharing your life with new and different people. These relationships will offer you positive, creative, and inspiring feedback from their perspective—and will ultimately influence yours.

Learn how to take one day at a time. Don't rush into new relationships and major life decisions too quickly, whether personal or professional. Preparing and planning for each day is great. Obviously, it is important to be as organized and as prepared as possible. However, as you transition, you need time to make changes and anticipating all of these changes is impossible! I soon learned that I was going through a period and change that I had never been through before and knew nothing about. I learned that you must accept each day, along with your accomplishments and contributions for that day! You cannot possibly know exactly what is ahead for you in this new period of your life. No matter how many people give you advice, it will not be enough to prepare you totally for each day and what it has to bring. I have learned to look at this positively and embrace it, especially on the most difficult days. It was the confidence that tomorrow would bring a totally new and different group of events in my life that got me through the toughest of days. I had to trust and learn that I could react with good judgment to the people and events presented before me each day and move on to tomorrow. Give time and thought to the new changes and relationships in your life. This will help you make the right choices for you.

Get to know who YOU are in this new phase of life. Learn your likes and dislikes, who you work well with and play well with, what you excel at, what you are passionate about, and your talents. This will be a process and may take some time. These things may have changed or may have been suppressed in your life. Learning who you are is important to making choices in life—including career, new friends, and new relationships in general. I certainly knew what some of my talents and likes were, but I have rediscovered a great deal about who I am. Some of it I have discovered from looking back at the past, some of it is from the new experiences and people I have met. I have grown and changed a great deal through this process. I have learned that I like to be surrounded with high energy people, those who are open to thinking outside the box, creative people, and people who are passionate about their work and lives. This has also been a very important part of keeping my life balanced and energized.

Over the years, I have made it a practice to contribute a portion of my free time to volunteering for various community, school, and church organizations. As I transitioned, I continued this involvement. It was a great use of some of my free time ,and I continued to know and see people that I might not otherwise have seen and connected with. I learned that I could have an impact on my community and in turn, my day-to-day life, by contributing and giving back. I have continued to become more engaged in my community's activities, both personally and professionally. I have learned to know more of my neighbors and what great people live in my neighborhood. I also have been able to keep in touch and learn what the needs are in the community and how I can help.

Lastly, learn to surround yourself with positive people in your life that will share the lifestyle goals and commitments with those you have set for yourself. Accept that you have to move on from time to time—from friendships and relationships—in order to get to the "right" ones for us. This may mean letting go of something or someone in your life. Also, please know this may be a process, but each relationship we have will help prepare us for the next. Having the right relationships and right people in our lives may take time but are well worth it.

In closing, accept the new and challenging phases and relationships that are set in motion for you. Be sure to take care of YOU as you transition through the new phases of your life. Reach out to help others—all of us have something to share and contribute!

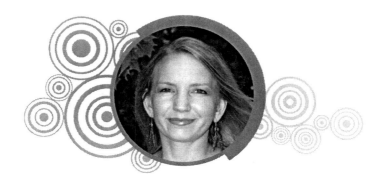

Sarah Mastriani-Levi, CHHC, AADP, RYT

Sarah Mastriani-Levi, creator of Mannafest Living, serves as an international holistic health coach and personal chef. She is often referred to as a boldly authentic spiritual pioneer, creative visionary, and inspirational catalyst. She lectures internationally and offers workshops and holistic health coaching for the health-curious to the avidly health-conscious. Parallel to her holistic consulting and various food services, she actively homeschools her four children, as a single parent, raising them with a strong bond to nature. She has raised them in an ecological manner, in harmony with nature. Her children have grown from all of the fresh goodness that nature has to offer, both physically and spiritually.

www.mannafest-living.com

- Skype: organic_veggie_girl
- contact@mannafest-living.com
- facebook.com/organic.veggie.girl
- facebook.com/MannafestLiving
- twitter.com/mannafestliving
- pinterest.com/MannafestLiving
- Sarah Mastriani-Levi, Personal Chef & Holistic Health Coach

CHAPTER 14

WHAT KIND OF VEHICLE IS YOUR VOICE DRIVING?

By Sarah Mastriani-Levi, CHHC, AADP, RYT

RENTAL CAR 101

Your body is a rental car.

You have been granted usage of this vehicle for all the days that you are alive.

When renting a car, there are certain elements that are usually "givens":

- It is going to be a newer car.
- It is going to be fairly dependable.
- There is going to be a backup service that you can contact in the event of an emergency.
- There are going to be massive fines to pay if you do not return the vehicle in the same condition that you received it, including the exact amount and kind of gasoline.
- These same rules apply from the lower-end models to the top models.

The equally important to mention "non-given" attributes are:

- Each vehicle is a "super-mobile" that Inspector Gadget could only fantasize about, with such amazing multi-tasking abilities.
- Each has the unique ability to regenerate itself, in totality every thirteen years. Yes, that's correct—you get a brand new vehicle every thirteen years.

The metaphor that our bodies are our vehicles is incredibly powerful. Your body is your vehicle, the house of your spirit. If not properly cared for, there will be steep fines that come in the shape of ill health and heavy medical payments. Pure foods fuel your vehicle. Keep in mind that you only get to use and enjoy this vehicle as long as you take care of it. Having a clean vehicle creates an unclouded environment, within which the spirit may take refuge and create a space for introspection and a place for spiritual growth.

The backup service that you once thought was only available "in the event of an emergency" suddenly becomes available intuitively on a regular basis. The moment you acknowledge your purpose and readiness to serve others, you discover that there is an entire support team rooting you on. There is no "right" way to be of service, other than to become aware of the special features that your vehicle has to offer. These special features are the different talents that are inherently available to whomever is willing to dig a little deeper to see what their vehicle contains.

How well you care for your vehicle is the message to the world of how they should treat you. When your vehicle has a clear direction and message, people notice the radiance and are inherently curious, respectful, and attracted. In spite of the fact that all of the vehicles came from the same "lot," not everyone chooses to bring awareness to everyday occurrences. Consistent awareness, coupled with fresh foods, fuels you to create a pure glow.

The moment this metaphor becomes a reality for you, you no longer are willing to fuel yourself with anything but clean foods. Eating this way over time enables you to create an unmistakably authentic voice. That voice is not clouded by misperceptions. Your voice becomes your purpose in life and your message is undeniable. The path is laid out before you, yet the journey of discovery is more important than the destination. In fact, the destination becomes irrelevant. The path of self-discovery and increased awareness creates the lessons we need to step into our greatness.

We must always remember that our vehicles are rental vehicles—we do not own them. The ego behind ownership has no place here. It can be taken from us at any point. It is a transient pleasure to use this body. The only requirements to continue using your vehicle are that you take care of it and that you show up and DRIVE. In spiritual development, no backseat driving is allowed. *Trying* is not sufficient. *Doing* is mandatory. When we *try* to do something that is not in alignment with our best direction, the universe has an amazing way of offering a lesson. If we fail to comprehend the lesson, the universe has a spectacular way of giving us the same lesson with different circumstances. Conversely, when we are following our right path, new roads are paved in our honor. Gratitude and satisfaction become permanent passengers along for the ride.

RELIGION AND SPIRITUALITY

> "We are not human beings having a spiritual experience.
> We are spiritual beings having a human experience."
>
> ~ Pierre Teilhard de Chardin

A spiritual practice really has nothing to do with religion. Religion is based on someone else's spiritual path to enlightenment. Individuals are inspired by that path and choose to become followers of a certain belief system based on that leader's experience(s).

Spirituality is creating your own experiences and belief system, and from those, deriving a spiritual path that serves to give your soul the opportunities necessary to shift your vision and come into alignment with your greater purpose. Religion and spirituality can both be present in an individual, yet they are not in any way dependent on each other for existence.

Are you being a voice or an echo?

The process of developing an individual voice can be quite daunting. There are so many messages out there, yet not one holds the magnificence of your unique voice. The process of discovering yourself, your spirit's purpose, and your voice is not an easy one. When one develops the desire to increase awareness, old belief patterns must be challenged. Do they still resonate with where you

COMPILED BY **MICHELLE GRANDY**

are going? Will they serve you in progressing or keep you trapped in a time warp of excuses, procrastination, and fear?

Fear and the belief of insufficiency undermine self-discovery and personal development on every level. The voices we hear that tell us in some way we are "not enough" are liars. They are echoes based on others' belief patterns and small-minded thinking. They have a primitive rationale that is designed to keep you safe. They scream, "Don't buck the system." Your potential to shine and create magic daily is greater than anyone could have ever led you to believe.

SPIRITUAL NUTRITION

Our bodies are built to serve us for the entirety of our time here on Earth. They radiate and innately carry a high vibration. Others sense this and are drawn to it. Intake of low vibrational foods, such as processed foods and animal products, slow down our vibration significantly. They limit our energetic potential as our body is so busy digesting. Our thought processes remain on a functional level and never really expand as long as low vibrational foods are consumed on a regular basis. It is as if we are giving mixed messages to the universe about our true intent.

Once a commitment is made to creating a lifestyle filled with more awareness, the universe speeds to respond in kind. Fruits and vegetables in their fresh, natural state have a very high vibration. They provide amazing energy, enabling us to step into our full potential of greatness. Vegan, vegetarian, and raw foods prove powerful tools in this process. Choosing to acknowledge the spiritual and energetic value of the foods we intake brings new meaning and relevance to creating a hearth that serves as an altar for feeding our spirits, and of those who share meals with us.

In conclusion, food is a sacred gift. Realization of that stimulates gratitude and honor each time we have the honor to consume it. Our bodies hold the potential to grow, heal, and change into vehicles of service. The cleaner our bodies become, the less encumbered our spirits are to create great change in our lives.

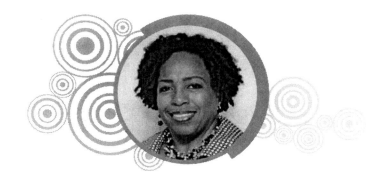

Denise Simpson,
MPA, CHHC, AADP, AAFP

Denise N. Simpson is an influential leader in the field of health and wellness. She is founder and CEO of My Life Healthy! with Denise, LLC, a company who is creating a movement of healthy living across the world. Coach Denise is a certified holistic health practitioner through the American Association of Drugless Practitioners, as well as a certified personal trainer. She holds both bachelor of science and master of public administration degrees from Florida State University. Coach Denise is married to her amazing husband Dennis of over thirty years, and is mother to three remarkable adults and "Grammy" to five wonderful grandchildren.

Are you curious about how Coach Denise's wellness and lifestyle coaching can help you?

www.MyLifeHealthy.com

f **facebook.com/mylifehealthy101**

W **Tumblr: mylifehealthy101**

📷 **mycoachdenise**

📌 **mycoachdenise**

🐦 **@mycoachdenise**

CHAPTER 15

EMOTIONAL WELLNESS

By Denise Simpson, MPA, CHHC, AADP, AAFP

Have you ever wondered what life would be like if we didn't have to deal with our emotions? Hmmm, that's a thought! Isn't it intriguing how our emotions play an intricate role in the expression of our feelings, whether constructive or indifferent? Truth be told, every action or reaction we have can be traced back to a simple thought that connected with both our feelings and our perception of the truth.

We have numerous thoughts daily that are triggered through sensory—see, taste, touch, hear, and smell—and memory perceptions. However, given the physical complexity of what's happening inside our heads, it's not always easy to trace a thought from beginning to end. The steady flow of thinking creates a constant network between our thoughts and feelings—our head and heart. No wonder we experience the proverbial emotional roller coaster—happy one moment, sad the next.

How we feel about ourselves, our environment, and our past experiences—whether good or bad—plays an intricate role in how stable we are emotionally. Depending on how traumatic our life experiences are, we can find ourselves trapped underneath the weight of emotions that we haven't fully dealt with. It's understandable that some experiences may be too painful to process mentally so we suppress the memory instead. The mind is so intelligent that it helps us cope with unpleasant experiences by filing them away in our minds until we are ready and willing to deal with them.

It's difficult going through the emptiness of being alone; the trauma that comes from being abused; being mocked as a child; experiencing betrayal or distrust in a relationship...all of these are real life experiences and there are many more—some with greater severity than others, but they all produce lower energy thoughts in our heads that connects with our emotions. The more we avoid closure, the more embedded the experience becomes within our subconscious mind, taunting us in one way or another and causing even greater anguish—excessive anger, self-sabotaging thoughts, feelings of inadequacy, fear, and anxiety attacks, to name a few.

So how would one go about breaking the cycle and reaching some level of stability or peace, if you will? Even though what I've described might seem like a downward spiral into despair, emotional wellness can be obtained. It will require patience and diligence to start the healing process from the inside out. And don't be afraid to get help if you need to. Sometimes all you need is the opportunity to express your feelings in a place that's comfortable and safe, where you will not feel judged. A health coach is a great resource to reach out to for guided assistance and for starting the healing process.

Healing begins with how you deal with your thoughts. Often we know when we are having a random surface thought as opposed to something deeper. But when it happens, think about how the thought came about. What triggered the feelings you are having? Was it something said or how it was said? Perhaps it was simply listening to a song? Ask questions of yourself, inquiring within as to how you feel about it and why. Continue asking yourself why until you get to the root cause of what you are feeling and why you are feeling that way. I call this peeling the onion.

I will be vulnerable and share a chapter of my life. The poised, confident woman that I am now has not always been. Through most of my childhood, I grew up not fitting in with most other kids. I was a loner, so to speak—didn't have many friends, stayed to myself, and had a mean streak. I was plagued for years with insecurities, feeling inadequate among my colleagues, and had a serious comparison complex of matching my weaknesses with the strengths of others. I was addicted to words while hating them at the same time.

My internal dialogue was not feeding me good thoughts, although I longed for them. I wanted to be affirmed in my identity that I was OK. But no one knew of my secret because I hid it all too well. I also struggled with self-acceptance. The mental picture of what I wanted in my life did not match my reality. This went on for years until I finally grew tired of my disposition. I'm not quite sure when it happened, or even how, but I just knew it was time to start plowing through the web I had created. I longed to be free of my own deceptions and the distressing opinion of others.

I started with accepting that I am a woman, called by God to do amazing things despite the contempt of men who told me otherwise based on my gender. This was a big step and an enormous relief within itself. I spent much time in prayer, meditation, soul searching, and journaling. It's amazing what happens when you begin to focus. As I made strides to freedom, divine intervention caused individuals to cross my path, reaffirming me with powerful words that fed my spirit and gave me courage to believe in myself. From this I gained a very dear friend who I can talk to about anything! Through her wisdom and spiritual counsel, I have gained wisdom of my own and have learned much about mental focus and stability in relationships. Her words are forever imprinted in my mind: "Stop using your computer (mind) to process things without having all of the information." I confess. I was guilty of coming to conclusions about situations based on my own perceptions without considering the probability of error. Are you too coming to conclusions about circumstances without validity?

We are the gatekeepers of our soul. What we allow to enter becomes a part of us—sometimes forever. So I hold steadfast to this principle, "Control your thoughts and you will control your emotions and your destiny." Words are powerful and have creative ability! What we say becomes our belief and then the law of attraction is our reward. Our thoughts, will, and emotions control our destiny and are responsible for how we see ourselves, others, and the world around us. What we focus on with thought and feeling is what we attract in our lives.

To be emotionally well means to be attentive to our thoughts, feelings, and behaviors—both positive and negative. It implies the ability to be aware of and accepting of our feelings, rather than denying them, all the while, being optimistic about life and enjoying it despite its occasional disappointments and frustrations, understanding that we tend to learn and grow during periods of difficulties.

Is it strange that we engage in physical activity that stimulates and conditions our muscles and cardiovascular system but rarely think to apply the same discipline to conditioning our minds and emotions for wellness? Having a strong grasp on the mind-body connection is important to maintaining stability. Emotional wellness is all about perspective and taking the higher road of viewing life's ordeals, come what may. Now, of course, I'm not encouraging that we negate or overlook our feelings. I'm simply saying to feel the emotion, give thought to how and why you are feeling a certain way, then take adequate steps to put your mind at ease so your heart can remain at rest.

Perhaps your story is similar to mine and you too have been a victim of your own device. If these words resonate truth deep within you, understand that you too can find your release and be unapologetically *free*! Free to be authentically YOU! This means loving the skin you're in, owning your confidence, and feeding your mind positive affirmations about your self-worth and disposition. You are brilliant, you are loved, and you are accepted—just the way you are. You only need to grab the reigns of your life and truly become the person you want to be—doing what it is that you've always wanted to do. Spend time thinking about what you enjoy doing the most. This is how I found my way to becoming a health coach.

I learned that I was doing this all along but never knew that it was called that by name. Good nutrition and exercising has been something I've been conscious of and enjoyed since high school, but I struggled with my weight because I did not like myself inside. I fed my emotions comfort foods that satisfied me during moments of crisis, but it always resulted in total sabotage of my self-esteem and my appearance. Today, it feels good to be free. This is my truth and you will find yours too.

May these words be forever engraved upon your heart and mind:

"Watch your thoughts; they become words.
Watch your words; they become actions.
Watch your actions; they become habits.
Watch your habits, they become your character.
Watch your character; it becomes your destiny."

~ Lao Tzu

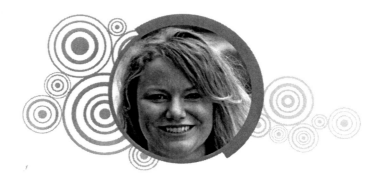

Elissa Kathleen, RYT

My name is Elissa Kathleen and I stand for love, authenticity, and possibilities in the world. I am an administrative assistant at DAL Global Services and a yoga instructor and trainer at Dancing Dogs Yoga. Most recently, I started my own business, Elissa Kathleen, teaching yoga, goal setting, and personal growth. I am a lifelong learner and believer in the power of intention. I challenge clients to go past their limiting beliefs, judgment, and self-doubt to achieve the things they say matter to them. "It is through radical self-love and acceptance that you become open to endless possibilities."

CHAPTER 16

FROM FEAR TO FREEDOM
By Elissa Kathleen, RYT

I'm not sure when I started doubting myself and being afraid to take action. It may have been instilled in me as a small child from church, experiences, family, or all of the above. I cared more about what people thought about me and I sought others' approval more than I checked in with my own true self. When I decided to write this chapter, I was scared. I almost didn't tell Michelle I was interested because it had me shaking in my pantaloons. I thought, "What if she doesn't want me to? What if I'm not good at it?" This is one thing I have been talking about doing since I can remember and now it is for always. I felt like, if I can share my experience with others, they can learn from it. If I can tell you how I overcame my own self defeat and did things I dreamed, maybe someone else would say, "Hey, if she can do it so can I!"

I have been on a journey of self and creating my path with awareness since my early twenties. My cousin, and best friend, talked about how we could make a difference in the world since we were little girls. As adults we decided we should write books to inspire women to help them see the facts and let go of the stories they made up about themselves. To have women see that no matter the odds, anything is possible. Back then, I got caught in the *how* of it all. I thought I had to write a 365-page book to have my voice heard. I was afraid to take the first step. What I have learned is that small steps turn into big results. I committed to this book as a small step, turning fear into action. I would love to tell you fear doesn't exist in me anymore, but that is far from the truth. What I can tell you is I don't let the fear run me. I acknowledge it, share it, give it up, take action, and repeat. Just saying it out loud, "I have fear and I am doing this because…," brings an opening for freedom. It brings an opening to do IT even if

I suck at it! Yes! It is OK to suck at something. You can't be an expert before you are a beginner. I remember learning to ride a bike when I was young. I would go over and borrow the boy next door's bike and ride up and down the street. I fell, over and over again. I sucked, but eventually I got it. Same thing happened when I bought my first car. It was a stick shift. I still think my neighbors laughed out their window while I stalled for twenty minutes at their stop sign, and my friends practically had heart attacks while I drove on 95, or stopped on hills, but I learned it. I'm no pro bicyclist or driver, but I'm good at. I'll tell you there are some things I am OK at sucking at, too. You don't have to be great at everything. What have you been holding back at doing because you are afraid to fail? What if you let yourself have freedom in trying something new, something that scares you?

My fears involved an underlying self-doubt that ran me. I didn't believe I was good enough for the things that I said mattered. When I met the owner of the yoga studio I work at now, I told her I had a yoga certification but wasn't teaching. She emailed and called and when I told her I didn't know how, she said, "You don't need to know how, just say YES!" I will never forget that conversation because it is how I ended up right here. I taught my first yoga class with a quivering voice, trembling hands, and full of self-doubt. Two years — and many classes, coaching, and self-inquiry — later, I now have found my voice and confidence to share myself authentically in the classroom and in life. I said when I first started teaching that I wanted to teach yoga trainings. I didn't know how, but I knew that yoga had transformed my life and I wanted to share it with others. Last month, I was asked and I accepted to teach a one-hundred-hour yoga training. So what happened next? FEAR! Once I committed and said, "YES!" the little crazy lady in my head started telling me, "You aren't good enough. It's not safe. You don't really want to do this." That's when I told myself, "Yes, you are good enough and you are a contribution." When I couldn't get past it myself, I reached out to my co-leader and got clear that it was normal and was able to move on. When I notice fear within myself, I think of it as a compass to tell me something matters to me. What matters to you? What are you telling yourself you aren't good enough to do? Where are you allowing your fear to run you? I challenge you to write down three places in your life you are choosing from fear. What would be possible if you chose from what is possible? Instead of making a list of all the things that could go wrong, what about everything that could go right? What about the lessons you could learn? What if you were willing to face your fear and be willing to fail?

I am facing that in my relationship right now. I realize that in every moment I have a choice. Up until now I have been coasting on comfort zone setting. I have been living my life going through the motions — work, yoga, husband, in that order. What I am realizing now is that I have put my relationship after others. I haven't been nurturing it to make it grow. My inaction has me in a place that I never thought I would be. I thought that my love was different. I thought we would thrive through everything. I realize I wasn't appreciating my husband for all he did. I was judging him for who he wasn't. I am afraid now our relationship will not recover. Now I have a choice to let go of fear and choose my love or to let it go. I don't have an answer for you today on my choice, but what I will tell you is I will be true to myself. I will make my choice from what I want even if I don't know how, because in the end anything that I want is worth the work. I never said that facing fear was pretty. Sometimes facing fear means taking a hard look at what isn't working and how you are responsible for it. It means looking at where your thoughts and intentions aren't aligned with your actions. What areas of your life aren't working? What can you do today to take a step toward what you want?

"When we are liberated from our own fear, our presence automatically liberates others."

~ Marianne Williamson

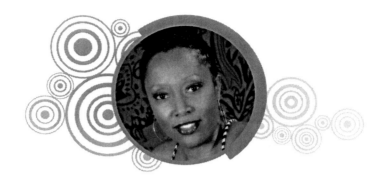

Angela D. Middleton, MEd

Angela D. Middleton is a skilled educator, trainer, visionary, and leader that possess a strong commitment to challenging and empowering people to be their best, whether they are in the classroom, workplace, or the community. She resides with her wonderful husband, Kendrick, and awesome son, Kyler in Oaktie, SC. She is passionate about taking care of those that God has allowed to cross her path. Angela believes that our purpose is to guide and build each other with our words and deeds.

Contact information:

✉ sah629@gmail.com

f facebook.com/angelad.middleton

in linkedin.com/pub/angela-d-middleton/4a/339/268/

CHAPTER 17

FAITH + PRAYER = IMMEASURABLE STRENGTH

By Angela D. Middleton, MEd

Angie,

"Arise, shine; for thy light is come, and the glory of the Lord is risen upon thee." Isaiah 60:1 (KJV)

I've always known this about you, from the first time our eyes met when you were born. I can't tell you how much I am so pleased with you and Shaun. We went through so much together, but that's OK, it is our path of life. The Bible tells us in Romans 8:28 (KJV), "And we know that all things work together for good to them that love God, to them who are the called according to his purpose." We don't know what his purpose is, but we do know that he has a plan and he will see us through.

So, be like the Virtuous Woman in Proverbs 31 (KJV). Be strong, kind, and loving as Christ is loving, keeping the faith through whatever comes your way. As James 1 says, "Count it all joy!" I have always told you, and I will say it again, put and keep God first in everything you do, no matter what!!!

I love you very much,
Moma "Momi"

What you read is the last letter my mom wrote to me four months before she passed away in February 2013. Mom was diagnosed with lung and bone cancer in June 2011. Her team of doctors did not expect her to live more than three months after she was diagnosed, but God had another plan for her so she lived 20 months longer than they expected. Cancer did not control her life or take her life, but it allowed everyone that crossed her path to see God at work.

The day my mom was diagnosed with cancer, she sat at the dining room table (our family's meeting place) and said, "I taught you all that there are consequences for your actions, good or bad, and this is the consequence of years of smoking." Her words were an avalanche of boulders that crushed me, leaving me breathless and trapped. A million questions surged through my mind like flashes of lightning across a stormy night sky. She immediately saw the anguish in my face and said, "But God is not through with me yet! I still have work to do." This "illness," as she referred to it, would be the test of my entire family's faith and our abilities to pour our hearts into our prayers. But the most valuable experience was watching God work through my mother, who battled crippling pain and fatigue, lifting people's spirits through prayer and counsel. Friends and family would come to visit her to encourage her and lift her spirits, but they found a woman with a smile on her face, a scripture to share, and a prayer for them that left them uplifted and prepared for whatever they would face.

Edwinia H. Gadsden—our mother, a wife, a sister, a friend to many, and a soldier in God's army—was my first spiritual teacher. She taught me that faith is believing in the Almighty God that created each one of us in his likeness, created the world that we live in, and has planned our lives from our births to our deaths. She taught me that prayer is thanking God for our lives and all of the things we experience, good and bad. She also emphasized the importance of praying for those who walk this path of life with us, because we are all on this path together, working toward the same goal—and that is to one day be with him and live an eternal life. Daily, my mom would spend time with God. It consisted of reading her Bible, prayer, meditation, and sharing God's love with everyone she encountered. She instilled in us that our minds and spirits needed to be fed daily by God in order for us to know what our daily purpose is and to live a healthy and productive life.

My mother shared her experiences in life whenever the opportunity presented itself. The words that she spoke and wrote were poignant.

I watched my mom battle cancer with dignity and immeasurable strength, while standing on the promises of God and drawing her strength from her faith in Him. Daily, I would hear her say, "I trust you, Lord," as she thanked him for allowing her to live and enjoy her life one more day. She reminded me that God makes no mistakes and that we should always allow his will to be done without questions, and to continue to do what he has purposed us to do. When stress would overwhelm me, she would reflect on some of the most stressful experiences in her life and say, "The things that are worth having require you to work hard for them! Remember, God will not allow you to carry more than you can bare, and don't forget Philippians 4:13, I can do all things through Christ which strengtheneth me." (KJV)

On Sunday, February 3, 2013, I said farewell to my first love, my teacher, my best friend—my mom. As we surrounded her bed in the house that my family had shared amazing memories in, I watched a peace that transcends all others wash over her delicate and tired face. At that moment, if I had never felt it before, I felt God's love pour over everyone standing in that room. She said to me a few days before she passed away, "Don't forget me." I grasped her hand and looked in to her eyes and said, "I will never forget you! Every time I speak, I hear your voice, and when I look in the mirror, I see your face. I am you and you are me." Although she is not here physically, I feel her love and embrace daily. Her lessons on faith and prayer have brought all of us through some challenging yet valuable times. This is the lesson that I am sharing with you, "Faith + Prayer = Immeasurable Strength." The beginning...

"For I know the plans I have for you," declares the Lord, "plans to prosper you and not to harm you, plans to give you hope and a future." Jeremiah 29:11

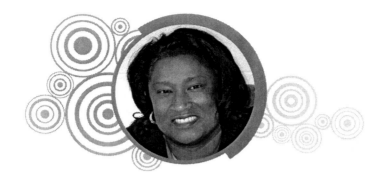

Gena P. Taylor, MPA

Gena, a native of Savannah, Georgia, lives a joyful life filled with the excitement of family and friends. She has spent most of her career in nonprofit administration and is currently the executive director of Greenbriar Children's Center. She's an experienced grants writer, evaluator, and professor. Gena has achieved many "firsts" in her life—first person in her family to earn a college degree; first African–American vice president of United Way of the Coastal Empire; first African-American coastal director of Lutheran Services of Georgia; and first African-American female of a rotary club in Chatham County, Georgia. Gena enjoys traveling, reading, and coloring.

CHAPTER 18

FIRST GEAR

By Gena P. Taylor, MPA

For me, any time in my life that I have had to shift my vision, it drives me to my core, to my center, to my foundation, to my faith. For it is in Him that I live, I breathe, and I have my being. Any time that I am making a life-alternating, life-changing decision, I have to make the shift first in my spirit and in my mind.

This writing takes me back to a very fond memory of my mother. At the age of five, I was baptized. I remember it was a winter day. Though the baptism was amazing, what was most amazing to me that day was my mother's joy as we walked home from the baptism. I could feel her love in the way that she held my hand, and I could hear the joy in her voice as she sang all the way home that day. I may not have understood the biblical meaning of baptism at that age, but in my spirit and in my mind I knew it brought joy and it meant love. My second baptism was different, in that I was an adult and my mother was deceased. The second baptism, while it meant joy and love, also meant newness.

I grew up churched. By the time I was ten years old, both of my parents were deceased and we went to live with my grandparents. They both attended Baptist churches but went to different churches. On the first and third Sundays, we went to church with my grandfather, and on second and fourth Sundays, we went to church with my grandmother. I remember the days of 2:00-6:00 p.m. communion Sundays, vacation Bible school, Wednesday night Bible study, Easter speeches and Christmas plays, and singing in the youth and young adult choir. I was churched. I remember my grandfather during his Sunday morning shaves, sing-preaching (no, he was not a preacher; not an ordained one, anyway), but it was all in preparing for Sunday service. If we did not watch television any other time as a family, we watched the Billy Graham crusade. I was churched.

What happened? Why is it that when I went off to college, I attended church probably four times of the four years that I was away? Of course, when I came home for weekend and holiday visits, I attended church. How is it that a person who had been churched as much as I was would want to go anymore? I observed this young woman in our church who appeared to have something more, but how could that be? She and I attended the same church and participated in the same church activities, but there was something different about *her* church and *my* church. As I mentioned earlier in this chapter, at five years old, you do not always understand the meaning of certain biblical principles, but as an adult, twenty-two years later, I was beginning to understand that there needed to be a shift in my spirit and in my mind first in order to create newness and lasting change in my life.

It was probably about four years ago when I had a shift in vision for my life. I wanted a more healthy life. I made the decision to run in the 2011 Rock 'n' Roll marathon/half-marathon. I of course was running the half-marathon: 13.1 miles. My commitment level was training for a span of twenty-four weeks. I would rise every Monday, Wednesday, and Saturday mornings at 5:00 a.m. to meet the other trainees at 6:00 a.m. I was feeling good because this was the first time I had done any type of running since 1979. You know I had to feel good about proving to myself and to the naysayers that, yes, at my age I could do this. I was looking good because I had lost a few pounds during the process. I was writing about my experience (writing always makes me feel good). When family and friends realized that I was serious about this, I must admit they began to inspire me in any way they could. Family members were excited because this was the first time someone in the family had attempted a feat such as this. My energy, confidence, and work productivity was at its apex. I recall running day—the adrenaline was rising with every step to the starting line. There was so much enthusiasm and energy among the walkers and runners. People on the sidelines were cheering you on and the bands kept you pumped. My training was proving to be essential to my finishing the half-marathon run successfully. As brutal as the run was, the moment I stepped over the finish line, I was already planning my running strategies for 2012. Victory was mine. I had done it and got a medal for it. I remember even dancing around the park after the run. I was happy.

Then Monday morning came and the "thrill was gone, baby." What happened? As good as the preparation for the run made me feel and look, I should have had a *new* normal, but instead there was a cessation; worse than that, I had reverted. It was as though the training and the run had never occurred. Guess what? I realized all of my energy had been about creating a critical mass for the run, but once I reached that tipping point, I really had no plans for maintaining or exceeding, so I reverted to what was comfortable and known to me. I actually became depressed. Can you imagine having that kind of success and then becoming depressed after? My diet was poor. I was not exercising, was watching all kinds of craziness on television, and became a hermit. I went for my annual physical exam and labs. When the results came back and indicated my cholesterol was high and I was pre-diabetic and the doctor began to write prescriptions, all I could think of was the bag.

What is the bag? The bag is the medicine(s) that our loved ones have attached to them as if it is a part of their body. It hurts to my core, each time I see one of the women who helped rear me now carrying bags of medicines. These were once very vibrant women with so much joy, courage, and strength; women who taught me to be Christ-centered; who challenged me to be the best I could be; phenomenal women. When the bag thought entered my mind, I instantly decided within my spirit and my mind that this was not the will of God concerning me. The Bible tells me that God "has plans to prosper me, not to harm me; plans to give me a hope and a future." I have resolved that I am worthy of this promise. I am not even a fan of roller coasters, so why was I riding one that was bearing my health as its name? I told the doctor there was no need to write the prescriptions because I would not need them. I left the doctor's office more determined than ever to own a healthy life.

Being healthy is more than the high of winning a medal, but it encompasses the whole being—beginning with your spirit and mind. If those two things are healthy, then a shift to a healthier body and lifestyle is imminent if you pursue it diligently. My daily ritual includes morning and evening Bible study and prayer, a consistent exercise program, and a healthy diet of fruits, vegetables, grains, and meat. I find that when I begin my day with prayer and exercise, it sets the tone for my day. I am much more energetic, productive, have a positive attitude and am much more engaging. I am more prepared to tackle the issues of the day. I have also taken the steps to alter my sleeping patterns so that I am getting the appropriate amount of rest. I did not realize how necessary adequate sleep is to a healthy lifestyle. I am much more watchful of what I allow into my spirit, as well. My appetite for television has shifted dramatically, and as a result of that, I find that reading is much more appealing to me. I find it helpful to have a mentor and a life coach (and could be the same person). This is a person I can trust, that challenges me and holds me accountable. It is also important for me to have a social life outside of work. I need time to play and enjoy life. Are there times when I "fall off the bandwagon"? Absolutely. The one thing I know and can and will do is to begin again the next day.

Whenever I need to make a life-changing, life-altering shift, it begins with my foundation, my core, my center, my faith…*first gear* for me begins in my spirit and in my mind.

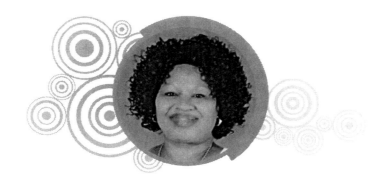

Carolyn Eiland, ANP-BNC

Carolyn Anthony-Eiland is a native of Savannah, Georgia. She is the daughter of the late Mr. Elmore Anthony, Jr., and Walking Deacon Rose Anthony, and is also the oldest of four siblings. She is the wife of Deacon Jerrell Eiland of twenty-five wonderful years, and the two are proud parents of four children—Dewayne, Jessica, Ashley, and J. Taylor.

Carolyn is a 1980 graduate of Sophronia Tompkins High School. She received her collegiate education at Armstrong Atlantic State University. She received an associate's degree in nursing in May 1994, and in May 2000, she received a bachelor's of science in nursing and the Don Levitt award for outstanding BSN student and a master's of science in nursing with a specialty as an adult nurse practitioner in May 2007. In 2007, she was inducted into the Sigma Theta Tau International Nursing Honor Society and board certified through the American Nurse Credentialing Center (ANCC). She is employed with Curtis V. Cooper Primary Health Care, where she's served dually as the director of clinical services and an adult nurse practitioner for twenty-two years. Carolyn is also a certified facilitator and core-lead for the Canyon Ranch Institute, Savannah.

CHAPTER 19

THE GATEWAY TO SUCCESS IS THE CONNECTION BETWEEN ONE'S SPIRITUALITY AND THE MIND

By Carolyn Eiland, ANP-BNC

Gateway is defined as an opening or entrance, or a means of access. Moreover; *success* is defined as a person or thing that achieves desired aims, attains fame, wealth, etc. — as defined by the Oxford Dictionary. When we look at both definitions, they reveal to us the importance of our spirituality and our mind being in balance. What is spirituality? Spirituality is the quality or state of being concerned with religion or religious matters: the quality or state of being spiritual. However, spirituality to me is having a personal relationship with God. It's intimacy with the eternal God.

At a very young age, I was always curious about God, nature, death, life, and how things came about. Because my father was a student of the Bible, which is the written word of God, and my grandfather was a man of much prayer, I spent a lot of time with both of them and would ask unusual questions concerning the things of God. There was always a longing to know more about God. It was almost like an inner longing or pulling for more of God. For me, the gateway and the access were always there, even as a child. However, the pathway was altered because my mind was fixed on the things of this world and not on things that were eternal.

Growing up in the inner city of Savannah, Georgia, in a community that was very close knit and a family that was not only close but was competitive, had high moral standards, and in a household with a mother and father who sheltered my siblings and I and didn't teach us or allow us to learn the street life.

I wanted to be a nurse by profession, but I didn't think I was smart enough to become one, therefore, I settled and decided to become a social worker to help people. But then college became the gateway to dating and partying, and I only did what was required of me to get by and still complete college. My junior year, I started to date a guy introduced to me by a good friend, and eventually that relationship became an abusive one. It lasted for six months, but to me it felt like a lifetime. At the end of six months of being physical abused, it seemed like there was no end. He followed me to school, waiting in the parking lot after class. And because a fear for my life was ignited, my professors had to walk me to my car. He was a shadow, and no matter where I went he was there to remind me that if he couldn't have me, no one could. In the spring of my senior year in college, my life changed forever.

In April of 1986, I was fed up and tired of being scared and took matters into my own hands. Unfortunately, I was arrested for involuntary homicide. I was devastated. My family was devastated. I had never been to jail. My parents had sheltered me. How would I ever survive this tragedy? It was my spirituality and my mind that would get me through six months of the county jail and six months of prison.

The gateway to my success was without a doubt my personal relationship with God and my mind. I thought that life for me was over, because I had become a statistic; the one thing that I never wanted to become. The jail and prison medical personnel tried to give me medication to keep me calm, but I refused them all.

My parents got the prison chaplain to give me a King James Bible, which would become my best friend, and I also began a prayer life. I would read it day and night. One of the first books I read was the Book of Romans, and I would meditate on Romans 12:1-2. "And be not conformed to this world: but be ye transformed by the renewing of your mind, that ye may prove what is that good, and acceptable, and perfect, will of God."

I had to disregard every negative thought that would come to mind. The only way to do this was to renew my mind and put off all negative and corrupt thinking and put on "God's thoughts." I began to learn that this process was the beginning of a true *over-comer*. "Overcoming" simply means freedom from self, freedom over circumstances, and freedom from others' responses. The bottom line was that having a renewed mind, putting off my own negative thoughts, and putting on the "mind of Christ" was the only way I could begin to see everything that happened to me from God's perspective and not get buried by my own thoughts. That gateway led me to understand that God had a plan for me before the foundation of the world and this plan encompassed the gifts and talents and desires that were burning on the inside of me.

In April of 1987, my father, mother, and siblings picked me up from prison and I can still hear my father say to me, "Carol, we serve a God of a second chance. Remember that He has a future for you." Before leaving, the chaplain at the prison gave me these words, "Better is the end of a thing than the beginning of a thing." To me, because my mind was renewed, these words were a breath of fresh air. God would, over the next couple of months, continue to divinely order my steps. I recommitted my life to Christ and continued to seek him through fasting and praying. In August of 1987, I met Mr. Jerrell Eiland. However, we did not enter in to holy matrimony until January of 1989. The gateway then led to the desire to fellowship with the local assembly. I joined the Owens Temple First Christ Holiness Church under the leadership of Orbert Harden. I began to grow spiritually and become an active member of the church.

The gateway was continuing to lead me to embark on the career I'd wanted as a child and that I didn't think I was smart enough to pursue. I enrolled at South College to become a licensed practical nurse, and in one year I graduated with high honors as salutatorian and gave birth to my first child, Ashley J. Eiland. In the fall of the next year, in 1991, I went back to college and received an associate's degree in nursing. In 1992, I graduated as class president and accepted a PRN floor nursing position at Curtis V. Cooper Primary Health Care, Inc. In December 1994, I gave birth to my second child, Jerrell T. Eiland, and accepted a full-time position at a Curtis V. Cooper Primary Health Care, Inc. public housing site as RN case manager, and later became the nursing supervisor of the site. In 2000, I received a bachelor's degree and the Don Devitt award for outstanding BSN student from Armstrong

Atlantic State University. In 2005, I enrolled in the graduate program at Armstrong Atlantic State University, and in 2006, I was inducted into the Sigma Theta Tau International Nursing Honor Society. I graduated in June of 2007 with honors with a master's of nursing with a focus specialty in adult primary health care and became board certified through the American Nursing Credentialing Center. In 2011, I was promoted to clinical practice manager and transferred to the main site at Curtis V. Cooper Primary Health Care, Inc. In 2014, I am now the director of clinical services at CVCPHC. My primary role is to oversee all clinical department supervisors and lead personnel, i.e., nursing, pharmacy, radiology, laboratory, and medical records at all sites. Recently, I was certified as a core team lead facilitator and intercreative health core team member to do one on ones through the Canyon Ranch Institute life enhancement program.

In the midst of God divinely leading, sometimes walking, and other times pushing through the gateway in the things of the natural, He was also pulling me closer to Him. My personal relationship with God kept me balanced. My mind was being transformed daily into the image of Christ, my words were his words, and I continued to decree and declare his plans and promises over my life. God was allowing my life to line up to the world. I was learning the answers to the questions I had as a little girl concerning God, life, death, and creation.

I could now see and clearly understand Jeremiah 29:11, KJV. "For I know the plans I have for you," declares the LORD, "plans to prosper you and not to harm you, plans to give you hope and a future." The NIV states, "For I know the thoughts that I think toward you," says the LORD, "thoughts of peace, and not of evil, to give you an expected end."

God was training and making a leader; he took me from the choir, to the missionary board, to the youth department. In 1994, my spiritual father went home to be with God and my spiritual mother became the apostolic leader, Apostle W. B. Jefferson. I have been sitting under her tutelage and under her leadership, ordained minister, currently, Elder Carolyn Eiland and serve as co-pastor of the New Greater Owens Temple Ministries, Inc.

Was it the family that I was born into? Was it all academics? Was it a magic formula? Was it simply who I knew? Was it being in the right place at the right time? The answer to all of the above, in my opinion, is no. It was the plan that He had for my life and making right choices even after making the wrong choices. Furthermore, if you follow the Holy Spirit and you allow Him to transform your mind. The healthy Connection of the Spirit and the mind will lead you to success.

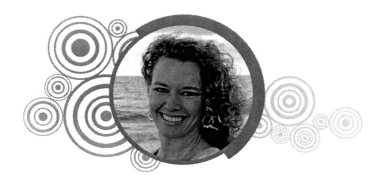

Holly Matteo, D.C.

Dr. Holly Matteo is a Christian, a mother to three children, a wife, and a chiropractor. Together her and her husband own and operate Matteo Family Chiropractic with two office locations: Bluffton, SC, and Hilton Head Island, SC. Dr. Matteo holds two bachelor's degrees— one in biological science from Rutgers's University and one in human biology from Logan College of Chiropractic. She also received her doctorate in chiropractic from Logan College of Chiropractic. Dr. Matteo's approach to patient care is unparalleled—she listens to the patient, looks at the body as a whole, and spends thirty minutes with every patient.

www.matteofamilychiropractic.com

www.twoorganicdoctors.com/

www.lifewave.com/twoorganicdoctors.com

f facebook.com/MatteoFamilyChiropractic

🐦 twitter.com/drhollymatteo

📌 pinterest.com/drhollymatteo/

in linkedin.com/in/drhollymatteo

CHAPTER 20

WOMEN AND CHILDREN

By Holly Matteo, D.C.

When I was young, my brother—who is four years older than me—was diagnosed as being hyperactive. My mother must have been on a mission to help her son because I grew up on the Feingold diet (http://www.feingold.org). As I was growing up, I noticed I ate different foods than my friends. My Easter baskets were not filled with the same junk as my friends' baskets, and my lunch box was plain. I remember on Sundays we were allowed Breyer's ice cream, and at dinner a small glass of 7-Up. My world was different; full of all natural foods with no dyes, chemicals, or fillers, but honestly, I didn't know exactly why this was so important. I just ate the foods my mom cooked and didn't question it. When I look back, it must have been a complete challenge for my mom. She was young, working, and planning healthy meals while her friends talked about the new convenient, pre-packaged food that was appearing in grocery stores in the 70s.

Around the mid-eighties, I started noticing a few "junk" foods in the pantry, like Tasty-cakes or diet soda, which was never there before. I can remember being about twelve or thirteen when I started having fainting spells. My mom called my uncle, who is a chiropractor, and discovered that the diet soda was causing me to black out and faint because of the artificial sweetener. So I immediately gave that up and never fainted again. Things around me innately started to click, and I was intrigued by chiropractic. I had no idea what chiropractic actually was, but I started telling everyone I was going to become a Chiropractor.

I went through high school with the same intentions, and my mom started working in a chiropractic office. My uncle lived across the bridge in Philadelphia and we were in South Jersey, so I had started chiropractic care with my mom's boss when I was fifteen. Why would a healthy fifteen year old need to go to the chiropractor? Simple, because I walked funny, and I knew it made me look awkward. That's the simple teenage answer! But I truly did have a hip issue and we discovered I was born with an extra vertebra. As a result, my spine didn't have the curves it's supposed to have. So why not take care of it on a regular basis to prevent any problems later? But as a teenager, I just knew it felt good and that I was walking more naturally.

Time went on, and as I started college, I became an EMT. During those years, I would work on Friday night and then wake up for the 4 a.m. shift on Saturday morning. During a shift one day, I slammed my head in the back of the ambulance so hard it caused me to black out for a few seconds while pain shot down my arms. After this happened, I went straight to my chiropractor and also to see my uncle. I started having severe migraines at this time, too. I was diagnosed with post-concussive syndrome. Severe mood swings and migraines would haunt me for a couple of years. But each time I got adjusted, I would get a little better, so I knew I was in the right place.

I graduated college and moved on to chiropractic school in 1997 with my high school sweetheart, who was also enrolled in chiropractic college. I hadn't been there a year when I was sitting in cell biology class and the professor was talking about birth control and how it stays in the liver eleven years. It dawned on me that the birth control was causing my hormonal migraines, and I needed to get off it immediately. It also occurred to me that maybe this is why so many women are having problems getting pregnant, since it takes so long to clear it out. For me, the hormonal migraines stopped immediately, and my passion was ignited.

After graduation, we got married and started our practice together. Even though I had cut out all junk food during school, we still decompressed with a few drinks on the weekends, so when I graduated, I was fighting an uphill battle with my weight. I began walking, running, and doing Pilates. I dropped twenty-five pounds and felt great. I was fresh out of school and thought I was rich with knowledge as a holistic doctor. Then one day during a big kids' event we were putting on with spinal checks, balloon making, etc., I noticed I felt very tired. I took a pregnancy test and it was positive! This is where my holistic journey began. Pieces of the puzzle kept on hitting me in the face; everything I had ever experienced had happened for a reason and I credit God for leading my mom in the direction of food with my brother's hyperactivity. Next, I became a reading and listening junkie about natural birth, and my main goal was to have a birth plan and live by it. I became interested in yoga and practiced yoga every other night. I walked and did Pilates through my entire pregnancy. Everything was awesome until I called my mom at our office (she worked for us in the office) from home and said I think I'm leaking amniotic fluid. A few hours later in Savannah, Georgia, I was told my water had broken and my baby was going to be born five weeks early. The OB immediately started talking Pitocin and an epidural. My face turned white; I couldn't believe my dreams were crushed that fast. My husband stepped in and said, "Wait a minute, we have twenty-four hours before it gets serious. Can we have time to do this without drugs? This was our plan." My OB looked at me and said, "You got it." Our goal was to maneuver this baby down the birth canal safely. So what's the first thing we did? My husband adjusted me right there in the OB office so my pelvis would start opening up more to let the baby drop. A quick trip to Walmart and we were in the hospital laboring on birthing balls, taking showers, and walking the halls. I had negotiated to have the fetal monitor on every hour and a half for twenty minutes but no other bed confinement. It was not perfect but, fourteen hours from start to finish and I had an all-natural birth with no intervention. My mommy instincts took over and although breastfeeding was a trial, I gave it time and it became easier and easier. Then organic baby food became my passion. At that time, my mother-in-law loaned me her Vitamix to make baby food. Eventually cooking whole organic simple foods became a passion. I have never once said any of this was easy and in fact, in the beginning, I was lonely and always felt like the odd ball around any women. All the moms I met breastfed for two months and then went to formula and gave their children baby food in a jar. Does this make it wrong? No! Most women, given the chance, would love to understand how to evolve into a mother that can do the best for her child or children. Medical mainstream, our government, Monsanto—they've all brainwashed us into thinking it's normal to take medication as a child or adult. This, instead of seeking chiropractic care to find the nerves that are causing interference and having the chiropractor help facilitate those nerves to fire again. In this country, it's normal to have cesareans without thinking of the baby's head molding that *should* happen when they go through the birth canal — because the mom was never properly educated on natural child birth. Or that it's normal to have food contaminated with pesticides and loaded with chemicals that are hidden in the labels using different names, which can causes allergies, ADD, behavior problems, diseases, cancer, suicide, etc. So my journey has never stopped. I had two more children naturally and kept learning more and more with each pregnancy. The journey has come full circle as I watch my children travel to the grocery store or farmer's market with me and learn about food, question drug commercials, and wonder why everyone doesn't see a chiropractor to keep healthy. My children don't know any better when they get sick. It's normal for them to get adjusted, use essential oils, have homemade bone broth chicken soup, and have homeopathic patches on acupuncture points. Moms have a responsibility to pass on so many things to their children, and many need to pull back and question why we are a nation of disease. Nothing is ever easy; it's a process and learning steps to keep a mom and her children healthy are imperative in today's world.

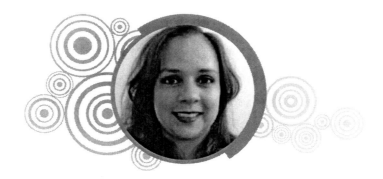

Janette Reyes-Heath PhD

Janette Reyes-Heath is a holistic nutrition coach with a PhD in arts of languages. She is also a Mexican-American and has studied in Mexico, England, and the US.

www.naturalgren.com

✉ **naturalgren@hotmail.com**

✉ **prof.jheath@hotmail.com**

f **facebook.com/naturalgrenllc**

🐦 **jheathealthy**

📷 **jennyreyesheathphd**

CHAPTER 21

INFLAMMATION

By Janette Reyes-Heath PhD

These days, we see so much food everywhere that all we do is mix and match what we see or think is healthy. Most of the time we're mistaken. All we are doing is saturating our gut with food that has a big impact on us. When you don't balance your foods correctly, you are susceptible to whole body "inflammation." This is fatal, as it affects our weight, lipids, glucose, aches and pains in your joints, headaches, and most of our internal organs, among others.

The best recipe for life to ease inflammation is to eat as much greens and vegetables and the rainbow colors in fruits every day. Of course, adding some grains, such as beans, lentils, and garbanzos—which are full of fiber—will also help.

I don't believe in diets but I do believe in optimal health that will make you feel gorgeous, radiant, with a better glow in your skin and less gassy and bloated stomachs.

Is time for you to love your body and give it what is craving for it? Just like your feet ask you every time for the fancy shoes, your tummy is asking you for the latest trend in healthy and easy food recipes that will make you feel un-bloated without constipation. As we say in Mexico, "Love starts with your eyes and ends in your stomach." Why? Because, first your eyes are delighted seeing all those delicious foods and then they end up in your tummy.

Most of the time we consume foods that trigger an adrenaline release, like carbohydrates, sugar, caffeine, etc. These foods boost energy for a short period of time but also increase glucose. When we consume food, we secrete some insulin and eating constantly contributes to "leptin resistance." This prevents the body from losing weight.

An easy remedy to ease body inflammation is to drink eight ounces of water with three tablespoons of vinegar. This will ease your inflammation and may help to low glucose and lipids. Take it before breakfast and dinner.

I practice what I preach, believe me. For years I've had to battle with several autoimmune diseases and hearing from medical doctors that "your pain is your head." Or "you are too young and I think you just want attention and some drugs." You cannot imagine how frustrated that made me feel. Even if it was understandable because I was a young preppy girl in her mid-twenties at the time.

I moved to California and as always, my husband went with me to the doctor's appointments. This time we went to a new rheumatologist. She said, "You know something, I think you have all those aches and pains you are complaining about because you are too fat." WHAT? Are you kidding? I responded so candidly, trying not to be angry. I told her that if I gained weight, it was because I couldn't move due to my pain and the aches in my spine, feet, and joints. I pulled out a picture and showed her. "I used to be Barbie and I am so sorry. Now I am Barney." I wanted to cry but I didn't.

I bit my tongue and continue listening to her and her opinions about my persona. My mind was wandering, thinking again how all of these doctors thought my pain was just in my head. She sent me to a back doctor and he put on me about three epidurals, but those did not work either. He said I have a tear but that he didn't know what's going on with me. We left his office and I was sad and frustrated, but I said to myself, "I will not give up because I know is something going on with me and God will send me in the right direction and find the right doctor."

All I can think is about the past and how I used to be very active and sporty. I ran almost every day, roughly 10 k. I was super thin had no problem with my health, until I was about twenty-five years old. After this age, I started having horrible joint pains, sciatica, and spine issues, among other things. It was very difficult and I could not move or continue to have the same type of active and sporty life I'd had before.

My quality of life began to go down dramatically and I started to have a sedentary lifestyle without much movement—all caused by joint, bone, and spine pain. And my eating habits suffered too.

I started eating more junk food, frustrated that no doctors believed me.

That's how I started gaining more weight. Add to that my inability to do any kind of sports or taking dance classes, Zumba, or aerobics. Just imagine, I was almost fifty pounds overweight at that point and felt like I looked like Barney on steroids.

Finally, one day I went to another new rheumatologist and he did a series of studies and a blood analysis and told us to wait outside. Time felt eternal and I felt for sure that it was another waste of time. Finally, after a few hours, we had the results of the studies.

The rheumatologist said to my husband and me, "I do regret to say that you have Severe Ankylosing Spondylitis and tested positive for the HLA-B27 gene. Also, you have rheumatoid arthritis, fibromyalgia, and Sjögren's."

Actually at that time, I was so happy that I almost danced. The rheumatologist put me on treatment, and even though I still have pain, it's not as strong as it was. I can say I finally do have some days that are better than others.

This is what made me want to study science in holistic medicine and holistic nutrition coaching—to help people like me. I have applied the same methods that I apply to my clients and I began to lose weight with a detox plan, anti-inflammatory diet, and a change of food habits. It was not easy but I am still following it. That's why I say: if I can do it, you can do it. Even when you see that the tunnel is all dark, remember, there is always a light at the end of the tunnel, and sooner and later somebody will hear you, take your hand, give you a hug, and say, "I hear you and I do understand your pain."

I'll be here to cheer you up and get you on the right path, no matter how many times you fall. We are humans and so therefore, we will have ups and downs—but you can do it. I know, I do not know what you must be feeling, but what I do know is that if you see me, it is because you related somehow with my story and that is a good start.

Because our health is invaluable and it is never too late to start taking care of ourselves.

Remember, inflammation accelerates aging and favors the emergence of many conditions such as obesity, hypertension, Type 2 Diabetes, depression, etc. And many studies have been made on the field of science about this. That's why I say, "No way, Jose!" I will not accelerate my aging process and conditions.

I am not telling you to put yourself in my shoes, but I do want you to put yourself in your own shoes and think about your health problems, and that new change you want to conquer. I know you can conquer everything you want because you are persistent. I know that many people—family members, friends, doctors, even co-workers—make you feel you have failed and they may have failed you as well, but you are the only person that knows what is deep inside and what you want to change—and how to shine the most.

Don't let your past define you. Let your courage, persistence, and present define who you want to b, and where you want to be in life. You have your life and loved ones that will be your motor to continue to run. Be grateful for every day—you can walk, jump, run, move, and dance, which is difficult for many people, including myself.

If you have that privilege, shine it! Be your own guide but also let yourself be guided when you need it.

Now, I'm happier! What about you? Now is time for you to be and feel happier. Please let me know if you want to be part of my journey and want to join some of my nutrition coaching and healthy classes.

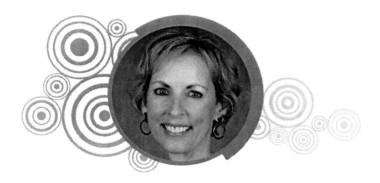

Julene Andrews, CHHC, AADP

Julene Andrews is a certified health coach passionate about "Designing Healthy Lifestyles." She inspires, educates, empowers, and supports others on their journey to become healthier and happier. She studied over one hundred different dietary theories through her studies at the Institute for Integrative Nutrition, and earned a certificate in plant based nutrition through eCornell. As a cancer survivor and two-time Ironman finisher, nutrition and fitness play a huge role in her life. Julene is dedicated to spreading awareness that by incorporating healthy, sustainable lifestyle choices today, we can impact our future health and live happy, healthy, abundant lives!

www.designinghealthylifestyles.com

✉ **julene@designinghealthylifestyles.com**

❶ **facebook.com/designinghealthylifestyles**

🐦 **twitter.com/andrewsjulene**

CHAPTER 22

WHAT LIVING WITH CANCER TAUGHT ME

By Julene Andrews, CHHC, AADP

"Whatever the present moment contains, accept it as if you had chosen it. Always work with it, not against it."

~ Eckhart Tolle

On August 18, 2011, my life took a major turn. I departed a plane in Phoenix where I'd just landed to take my daughter to her first year of college at Northern Arizona University in Flagstaff. It was an exciting time. Our oldest was a junior at the University of Idaho, and with our youngest leaving home, my husband and I would now be empty nesters. We were looking forward to this new time in our lives and had numerous adventures planned in the coming months. When we got down to the baggage claim, I checked my phone for messages. I had a message from my doctor back in Boise asking me to call her ASAP. Hmm, I knew this couldn't be good. When I called back and was put through directly to her, she proceeded to tell me a polyp I had removed weeks ago tested positive for uterine cancer. I was informed I needed to rush home for an emergency hysterectomy. I was in shock: I have cancer?

It was exciting for me to be visiting Phoenix again. Just nine months before, my husband and I had competed in Ironman Arizona, crossing the finish line together hand in hand. We were both in the best shape of our lives. We had always made choices to live what we thought was a healthy lifestyle. We both had professional careers, spent quality time with our two amazing children, and enjoyed spending free time running, biking, swimming, playing tennis, and hiking. As athletes, we ate what we thought was healthy: lots of lean animal protein, as well as drinking three glasses of milk a day. I had many people tell me I was the last person they thought would ever get cancer.

Upon returning to Boise, I met with an oncologist and learned I had a very rare and aggressive form of cancer. The prognosis was not good. In fact, he discouraged me from going home to look up the odds on the Internet. My question to him was, "How did I get this?" He answered, "You were just unlucky." I asked what I should do differently. "Nothing, you're doing everything right," he'd answered. He proceeded to tell me treatment would consist of surgery and then six rounds of chemotherapy over a four-month period of time. And yes, I was going to lose my hair. I had one more question for him. The signups for Ironman Canada were in three days and I was planning on doing the race with several friends. I asked, "Will I be able to do a full Ironman next August?" He looked at me in disbelief before answering. "Yes, I think you'll be able to do an Ironman next August."

My family and friends rallied around me with support. I was amazed at the many ways people reached out to us and blessed our lives. Throughout the time I was receiving treatment, I spent time training for Ironman Canada. There were days when all I could do was a walk around the block. But other days, when I had planned to meet friends for a workout, it proved to be a good distraction from the toll that chemotherapy was taking on my body. Race day came six months after I finished treatment and I lined up at the swim start with six friends from Boise. The entire day was like a dream; I appreciated the fact I was even there. I was healthy enough to race, my family and friends were there to cheer me on, and two of my friends were going to do the entire race with me. We swam 2.4 miles, biked 112 miles, and ran 26.2 miles, crossing the finish line before the midnight cutoff to hear the announcer calling our names and pronouncing, "You are an Ironman!"

During our stay in Penticton, Canada, my husband Steve noticed a nagging stomachache that wouldn't go away. We assumed maybe he had developed a kidney stone or had contracted a case of giardia. Upon returning to Boise, he went to the doctor and had some tests done. We were having dinner with friends before a Jimmy Buffet concert when Steve received a phone call from his doctor. He took the call and was told, "You have cancer." Unbelievable. Within the same year, both of us had cancer; I was diagnosed at age forty-nine, Steve at fifty-one. Neither of us had any previous health issues. How could this be?

In the months to come, we found out that Steve had Stage IV stomach/ esophageal cancer. In meeting with the oncologist, we learned the cancer had spread to Steve's liver, lungs, and lymph nodes. The prognosis was not good: He was given two months to a year to live. We left there in complete shock and deep distress. We had a decision to make: go home and die, or go home and live? We chose to go home and LIVE! We chose to stay positive. We turned our worries over to God. We reached out to friends for support. We both continued to work and do the things we love. Steve, despite having had twenty-four rounds of chemotherapy, competed in Ironman Boulder 70.3, and other triathlon races. We traveled and spent quality time with loved ones.

It has now been three years that we have lived with cancer. While they have been the hardest years of our lives, they have in many ways been the best years of our lives. Here is what we have learned:

- Life is short. Enjoy every moment. Appreciate the little things. Do today all of the things that you hope to do "someday."

- Focus on your blessings. Be grateful. Stop and be thankful for all of the good things in life. It's easy to dwell on the negative but if you can't change the outcome, why not forget about it and focus on the many ways you have been blessed. Bad things happen. It is what it is. Accept it, embrace it, work with it, and make the most of it. Choose to be happy.

- You are what you eat and drink. The Standard American Diet—which is high in animal protein, processed food, added chemicals, sugars and refined grains—is killing people. Your body needs plenty of water and the minerals, vitamins, and phytonutrients that are found in fruits, vegetables, legumes and beans, nuts and seeds, whole grains, and healthy fats. A whole food, plant-based diet will allow our bodies to fight the toxins we are continually exposed to on a daily basis.

- Other lifestyle choices matter. Disease thrives in a body that is not well cared for. Your healthy body needs an average of eight hours sleep a night, limited stress in your daily life, a minimum of thirty minutes of physical activity at least five days a week, healthy relationships, a fulfilling career, and a deep spirituality. All areas of life must be healthy in order for your body to fight off disease. Doctors say, given half a chance, the human body will heal itself.

- Don't ever give up. Stay positive. Some days are harder than others. On the tough days, just get out and take one little step in the right direction. Keep moving forward. Some days will result in a step backwards, but overall keep moving forward.

- Above all, trust in the Lord's plan. He has a plan for all of us, and while we might not understand why things happen the way that they do, we must learn to trust His plan. We grow and learn from our challenges.

There is inspiration all around us. We just need to keep our eyes open and look for it. I find it every day in my husband and children. Steve is the most genuinely happy person I have ever met. He never complains and finds the good in every person, situation, and day. I strive to be more like him. My son Michael is a lot like his dad. He, too, inspires me to be a better person. He is a friend to everyone he meets. He will be racing at Ironman Arizona this fall and has raised $5,000 in honor of his dad, to be donated to Debbie's Dream Foundation: Curing Stomach Cancer. My daughter Karlie is an inspiration in that she has never backed down from a challenge. She is a hard worker, set goals, and goes after them. And she makes time for more fun than anyone I know.

Going forward, my mission is to spread awareness that the majority of chronic disease is preventable through healthy behavior. My hope is to inspire others, and my passion is Designing Healthy Lifestyles.

"Life's challenges are not supposed to paralyze you; they're supposed to help you discover who you are."

~ Unknown

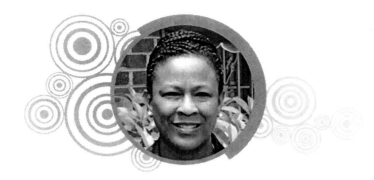

Lorna Jackson, DDS

Life was not easy for a young girl growing up in Biloxi, MS. I am the youngest of seven children. It is my belief we are all born with a gift. My gift happened to be my ability to run fast. I was recruited to attend Jackson State University on a full scholarship. My gift is the reason I received my bachelor of science degree in biology.

After leaving Jackson State, I decided to pursue a career in dentistry. I attended Tennessee State University Dental Hygiene School for one year, and after one, I was recruited yet again but this time to attend Meharry Medical School of Dentistry. Four years later, as class president, I received my doctor of dental surgery degree.

Coming from humble beginnings, I truly believe in my favorite scripture in Proverbs 3:5-6, "Trust in the Lord with all thy heart and lean not to thine own understanding, in all thy ways acknowledge him and he will direct your path."

CHAPTER 23

USING MIND AND SPIRIT TO STAY MINDFUL OF THE IMPORTANCE OF HEALTH/THE IMPORTANCE OF DENTAL HEALTH

By Lorna Jackson, DDS

Many people do not understand that your dental health can affect your mental and physical health. When you look in the mirror and smile, the first thing you notice are your teeth. Teeth come in different shapes and colors. Your teeth can govern the shape of your face. The basis of good teeth is the bone and gum tissue that holds them in. Periodontal disease is the destruction of these structures.

There is an old saying, "When you look good, you feel good." There are many ways today we can change the way we look when we smile. We can straighten our teeth with braces, we can whiten our teeth with different forms of whitening methods, we can change their appearance with veneers, and we can replace missing teeth.

Women have special oral health needs and considerations. Hormonal fluctuations have a surprisingly strong influence on the oral cavity. Puberty, menses, pregnancy, menopause, and use of contraceptive medication all influence women's oral health and the way in which a dentist should approach treatment. During puberty, we have an increase in hormone levels and this has shown a correlation to increased chances of gingivitis. Gums become red and inflamed. There may also be an increase in plaque and calculus deposit. Bleeding may occur when patients brush their teeth or eating. Oral changes that may occur during menses are much like the hormonal changes. There might be an increase in swollen red gingiva. And some have complained of bleeding and swollen gums in the days preceding the onset of menstrual flow, which usually resolves once menses begins. Other oral changes include activation of recurrent herpes infection, oral ulcers, longer bleeding following oral surgery, and swollen salivary and parotid glands.

The notion that pregnancy caused tooth ("a tooth loss for every child") and that calcium is taken away from the mother has no evidence. Calcium is not transferred in the circulatory system. How can oral health affect you and your baby? Pregnant women who have gum disease may be six times more likely to have a miscarriage or have a baby that is born too early and too small. Any infection during pregnancy is cause for concern. A mouth infection can cause low birth weight, putting your baby at risk for cerebral palsy, chronic lung disease, or even death. Hormones the body releases in response to labor may be similar to hormones released in response to infection.

During menopause, many women report a complaint of pain, burning sensation, altered taste, and dry mouth. Other conditions that can be related to oral hygiene are osteoporosis, burning mouth, Sjögren's syndrome, thyroid disorders, and oral contraception.

There is another old saying, "You can't build a house on quicksand." Periodontal disease is the quicksand of the oral cavity. Periodontal disease can range from mild gingival inflammation to serious gum disease, resulting in tooth loss and major destruction of gum tissue. Gum disease is caused by bacteria. Our mouth is full of bacteria. As a result of buildup, these bacteria form plaque. Brushing and flossing can remove this plaque, but if allowed to harden, plaque becomes a hard material called tartar or calculus. This can't be removed just by brushing or flossing. This has to be removed by a dentist or dental hygienist. The longer plaque and tartar stay on teeth, the easier it is for bacteria to lead to gingivitis, which cause swollen, inflamed gums. Gingivitis can be reversed with daily brushing and flossing and regular visits to a dentist. When gingivitis is not treated, it can advance to periodontitis, which means inflammation around the teeth. The tartar that is attached to the teeth causes a space between the teeth and the gum tissue, which becomes infected. Bacteria toxins and the body's own natural response to infection start to break down the bone and the connective tissue that holds the teeth in place. If not treated the bone, gums, and tissue that hold the teeth are destroyed. The teeth may eventually become loose and have to be removed.

Need a reason to quit smoking? Well, smoking is one of the most significant risk factors associated with the development of gum disease. Smoking can lower the chances for successful treatment. As mentioned before, hormonal changes in girls and women make gums more sensitive and make it easier for gingivitis to develop. People with diabetes are at higher risk for developing infection, including gum disease. Diseases—like cancer or AIDS, and their treatment— can also affect healthy gums. There are hundreds of prescription and over-the-counter medications that can reduce the flow of saliva, which has a protective effect on the mouth. Without enough saliva, the mouth is vulnerable to infection, such as gum disease, and some medications can cause overgrowth of the gum tissue that can make it difficult to keep gums clean. Gum disease can also be hereditary.

People usually don't show signs of gum disease until they are in their thirties or forties. Men are more likely to have gum disease than women. Although teenagers rarely develop periodontitis, they can develop gingivitis, the milder form of gum disease. Most commonly, gum disease develops when plaque is allowed to build up along and under the gum line.

Picture how close your teeth are to your brain. The distance is less than the size of your hand. An infection or abscess in the mouth can quickly spread to the brain. Twelve-year-old Deamonte Driver died of a toothache. A routine eighty-dollar tooth extraction might have saved him. The bacteria from the abscess had spread to his brain, doctors said. After two operations, and more than six weeks of hospital care, Deamonte Driver lost his life. According to NBC affiliate WLWT, Kyle Willis' wisdom tooth started hurting two weeks ago. The dentist told him he needed to have the tooth pulled. He decided to forego the procedure because he had no insurance. The tooth infection spread, causing his brain to swell. He died. John Schneider was thirty-one years old. His family thought he had a sinus infection and he was admitted to hospital. Doctors found out John Schneider actually had a tooth infection that turned into sepsis. He had open-heart surgery. He passed away.

President Theodore Roosevelt and President George Washington were both said to have dental infections that may have led to their death.

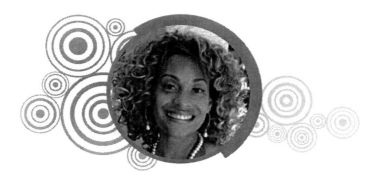

Candace Woodson

Candace Woodson is a professional singer, entertainer, and author. Candace began her music career at the age of five, with her musical roots in gospel. She graduated from Tennessee State University in Nashville, TN, with a BS in Commercial Music at Tennessee State University. After graduation, she went on to pursue a career in the music industry, receiving a recording contract. Her greatest accomplishment is raising her two sons to be young men with character. She is currently the lead singer of Candace Woodson and the Domino Theory Band. She resides in Hilton Head, SC, with her family.

 woodson_candace@yahoo.com

CHAPTER 24

RIDE THE WAVE
OF PASSION AND SUCCESS

By Candace Woodson

Careers—we all have one whether we like the one we have or not. Careers are determined by choice. A choice of following the path less traveled or the path that keeps me just like everybody else…"safe." The choice, believe it or not, happens in the womb. There is a plan for all of us. We are destined. The love of life helps your choices to fit your needs. One should not choose a career because everyone else is doing it or because it's easy. The choice of a career should be based on a desire to make a difference. Choosing the right career leads to entrepreneurship. They go hand in hand, and there are steps to follow. Little did I know, the gift God gave me at five years old would provide that bridge into entrepreneurship.

During my college years, the one voice that would not let my dream of being an entertainer die was the band director. He said, "You've got it!" And after auditions, I was selected as the lead singer for the college band. I was so happy because I thought, *Now I am on my way.* I failed to mention that once I graduated from high school, I received an offer to be in a band but turned it down. Achieving this honor to me showed that your gifts will make room for you. I ended up leaving that college after a year and enrolled in another one while working at the same time. I decided that the workforce was safer, and I became a training supervisor for a national shoe chain. They used me as the face of their product and another gift of my personality developed into building relationships for the future. I was constantly asked why I was selling shoes with a voice like mine. I knew I needed to eat and live, so the option of a music career seemed unrealistic. I thought it was impossible to live out your dream. How could I build a career and have it lead to entrepreneurship? In my opinion, I didn't fit the category of an entrepreneur. It finally hit me that all was not lost in being an entertainer when I took a final exam. Instead of writing it, I sung it and nailed it. It hit me that I really could do this if I tried. The keyword was *tried*. In the meantime, I started working for agencies and working in commercials, and also doing print work. I really believe you have to act *as if*. Thus this is the beginning of the umbrella effect. It was an eye opener. No longer could I fight the wave current of this path that had been set for me to embark on. I tried to have a career that was safe and what everybody else thought I should do. It's never the right thing to do as a career if it's only because others want you to—*you* have to believe. A career does not make you, you make the career. The career will lead to the entrepreneurship because wisdom and knowledge will be gained along the way.

I packed everything up and set out to prove to the world that this is what I should have been doing a long time ago. I was somewhat angry because I felt the world should have helped me more. I soon found out the world was not stopping me from achieving. The truth is, I was stopping myself. It was also easy to play the blame game with family and friends, but it is true what is for you is for you. How many times did I hear you need to get a real job? Job, not a career. When we realize there's a difference, then our mindset changes to face whatever comes with it.

This brings me to the significance of following the wave current of success. I moved once again and enrolled into a college for a third time, and yes, this third time was a charm. I was determined to get my music degree because when I made it, no one was going to say I was not qualified. I'd always worked jobs and tried to be a responsible adult according to society. Everything should be in Divine order. It is important to get under an umbrella because the rain is coming. You must stay covered as your journey unravels. You don't have to know everything, just keep trying. The enrollment into this college became the umbrella of foundation. Teachers, staff, and fellow classmates helped me and joined the charge of dreaming it. Thus is the process for building a career. A plan, education, hard work, passion, and having the skills is what makes a career.

Stepping in and out from under the umbrella wastes time. Why get wet for nothing? Staying dry protects you from things that you can't control. Don't be like those who say I'm going to do *this* but I'll have *this* to fall back on. You'll fall back every time. A career is born and goes through different developmental stages and you must weather the storm. You must look in the mirror every day and know who you are and confirm that your choices are spirited-filled. Tell God you want whatever He has to give you and know that His way is better than anything you can think of. Nothing is a waste of time!

In college I learned to sing and dance at the same time. I became polished. I stayed under the umbrella. Once I graduated I had the paper to say I was a part of the educated professional world. But there was still no music contract and all of my networking and projects seem to not prevail. So doubt set in—I wanted to follow tradition and get a job. Here is how the umbrella provides a shelter of protection. The Holy Spirit surrounds you and the comforter comforts you. A career is a faith builder and the experiences allow you to know who the author is of the experience. I went on to do radio, which lead me to a job at a record label. *Stay under the umbrella.* I managed the career for others, and I learned about the industry inside and out. When times were hard and I needed to find an income, I had a career. But now it was time to be an entrepreneur.

I developed a band and became my own boss. The *no's* didn't bother me. I'd heard them before. I was ready. The career created a *strength*. It's not based on one particular thing—it's everything. A job is a stagnated mindset where you're controlled not by dreams but someone else's insight and paycheck. With a job, you're not doing what you're called to do but doing what you're *told* to do. Once I removed myself from the workforce, I stayed under the umbrella that always kept me connected, using my God-given talent. It's the *something* you do that no one else like you can do. There is no explanation and no explanation is needed. The God-given talent builds the career, which will lead you to the entrepreneurship.

Remember the words of value you receive early in life. They are molding your thought process. Being rejected isn't always a bad thing. It can give you the push you need. Entrepreneurship is not forced. It is a laid-out foundation with a blueprint that has already been put in place. I am a firm believer that you can always have a career, but you can't have an entrepreneurship without a career being in place.

As for me, the journey was well worth it. A career is first and then the entrepreneurship that I own and I say own because the final step is ownership of it all. Under the umbrella it has created opportunities for me, such as becoming educated, acting as a radio personality, television host, and a manager and leader singer of a band. I am an entrepreneur *with a career*. Now, I can also add author to the list. Had it not been the foundation of ridiculous faith and relationships, I would still be wandering in the wilderness of hope and asking, who's going to fix this for me? Or what am I really put here to do? A career really does have purpose. Live it the dream, be it the dream, speak it the dream—all of it is a part of the final say so of achieving the ultimate goal career and entrepreneurship.

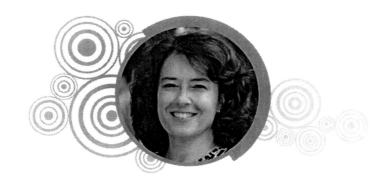

Lynette Becks,
RN, BSN, MPA, ERYT-200

Lynette Becks is a senior executive in the healthcare industry, has been practicing yoga since 2003, and has been a certified yoga teacher since 2009. She became a certified teacher for Baptiste Power Yoga in 2013. She is married with three wonderful grown sons and was happy to gain her first daughter upon her eldest son's marriage. She and her husband, Charles, also have three grandchildren who constantly amaze them. As a registered nurse and certified Baptiste yoga teacher, Lynette has a passion to assist others in opening a new universe of self -discovery and promoting health and positive well-being.

✉ lynette@dancingdogsyoga.com

CHAPTER 25

TAKING YOGA OFF THE MAT AND INTO THE CORPORATE ENVIRONMENT

By Lynette Becks, RN, BSN, MPA, ERYT-200

I have always felt that I did not find yoga but that yoga found me. I joined a fitness club to get back in shape and I went to attend my first aerobic workout but found a yoga class replacing it. I was all set to leave the club.

The yoga teacher stopped me and invited me to stay. I declined, giving all kinds of excuses. *I was not dressed right. I did not have a yoga mat. I did not know how to do yoga.* In actuality, I just thought, "No way, I cannot do that. I want to work out, not just sit still and say 'ohm.' What a waste of time".

I decided to stay and I was quite surprised. The class was very physical. It was constant flow and I broke into a sweat. So much for "ohm!" I fell in love with yoga and felt like I was coming home. It was exactly what I needed. It was a good workout and I felt calm after the class.

I have stayed with the practice for the past eleven years and have tried many styles of yoga. I always gravitated back to the more physical classes. Eventually, I found the style that truly resonated with me—Baptiste power vinyasa yoga.

Often, people think yoga is only a physical practice. The practice and techniques of Baptiste Yoga contain three elements—asana (the yoga poses), meditation, and inquiry. Practicing asana is thought to prepare the body to sit in a meditation position for periods of time. Inquiry is the looking within oneself to the way we think, react, and feel.

I found the physical practice invigorating. Getting sweaty with movement and heat brought me the ability to create stillness, both in my body and my mind. Tensions dissolve like liquid, dropping to puddles on the floor. My worries fell away.

As I reached a level of calmness in my body and mind, I was able to reflect on how I reacted and interacted with others. Through Baptiste Yoga, I read about *The Collaborative Way* by Lloyd Fickett and Jason Fickett. They discussed the Ethics of Responsibility and five core principles, which include listening generously, speaking straight, being for each other, honoring commitments, and acknowledgment and appreciation. These principles are a part of the yogic way, as well if you begin study on the Eight Limbs of Yoga.

As I reflected on my life off the mat, these principles resonated with me. I realized my life and everyone else's was about relationships—in family, in work-life, and in the larger community.

My way of being affects not only me but also everyone around me. I can and do make a difference in this world through my connections with others. I can be a positive contributor if I so choose. If I am a negative contributor, I am able to shift my vision and my attitude to the positive side. It is all within my own power and control. How liberating!

So, I chose to make a positive difference. With gratitude, I listen generously to others. I now listen more intently to what the other person is really trying to say and not what I want to hear or through my own filters. We all have already existing automatic listening aspects to our hearing. I identify mine, drop them, and truly listen to the other person. It is amazing how different the message can be.

In speaking straight, I flexed a new muscle to speak from my heart and not my head. If I want to say something, I say it truthfully but with added compassion. I have always prided myself on speaking the truth. What I needed to add was to look at what I say and how I say it—how it lands on others. It is possible to get my point across with kindness. What a difference it makes! The other person will most likely listen generously back and take in what I am saying rather than posturing defensively and considering their retort, not even hearing what I am trying to say.

Honoring commitments is so important because it is my word. How can I be taken seriously if I cannot be trusted? How can another human being trust that I will follow through with what I say if I do not honor the commitments I make? I find I often want to do everything (such a type A personality, I am) and then get myself in predicaments where I have way too much on my plate. I say yes to everything and then have absolutely no time or space for myself.

Honoring commitments for me is not just a practice in following through, it is a practice of acknowledging how much I have already committed to and giving my word for a completion timeframe that is realistic, rather than unrealistic or compressed. This in itself is liberating. I say when I can finish it, so why not set it to a date that I can truly manage! I used to be my own worst enemy with time. Now I am more realistic with myself and what I can accomplish, and on time.

 The practice of acknowledgment and appreciation is very interesting to me. Instead of just saying thank you, I now look the person in the eye and acknowledge what the other person has done and why it is meaningful. In the past, I rarely realized that my connections with others were superficial. I did not look others in the eye with regularity. I was looking forward to the next thing to do, to accomplish. Now I stay present in the moment and truly appreciate my connections with others and my relationship with others. It has been interesting to see how many others make these eye-to-eye connections. When someone looks at me, I think, "Wow, they really see me."

All of these practices also belong in the workplace. We are humans with feelings and responses at work, just as we are at home and in the community. Connecting with others in the work setting makes a difference.

Those I connect with at work are much more likely to understand what I am requesting and the why behind it. With understanding, the other person will follow through on the work activity needed. If there is a breakdown and something goes wrong, as a team we look at what went wrong and fix it. Most often it is a breakdown in process and not with the person. Taking this approach leaves both of us feeling empowered and in control of our actions. The goals of the organization then move forward.

Because this works so well, I introduced the Collaborative Way® to the management team that I oversee. Approximately fifty management team members are attending Collaborative Way® workshops. We have set up a buddy system for the team as they grow in their own yogi self-inquiry and exploration.

Has it made a difference? Absolutely! Before we began the Collaborative Way®, team members communicated through instant messaging (IM) and e-mail. Feelings would sometimes be hurt, misunderstandings occurred, and projects took longer to complete timely and effectively.

Now team members talk to each other and listen to what each and every person is saying by listening generously. If they do not understand, they ask questions rather than making assumptions. They talk in person or on the phone with a video camera on so they can see each other. E-mail and IM are used but not for items that require input from both people. No longer is it possible to hide behind the anonymity of technology. Relationships are important and they can be diminished with technology today.

Projects are completed timely and with deliberation. Perceived obstacles have faded away. Possible breakdowns are identified before they even come to fruition. This has made our work environment more effective and efficient.

The office is energized and the personnel can see a difference. Personnel see that their supervisors are not distracted and spend more time in 1:1 conversations with them.

Does yoga off the mat work? Does it work in the corporate work environment? Most definitely it does!

What are you waiting for? I invite you to get on a mat and come to a clear understanding of how you think, react, and interact with others.

If you are unable or unwilling to get on a yoga mat, you can still be a yogi off the mat. Take on the Collaborative Way®.

Today is all that we have. The past is gone and the future is not here yet. Make a difference today. It is worth it. You are worth it and your connections are worth it, as well. My teacher, Baron Baptiste, once in a class, said to *teach every day, and sometimes with words.* I have taken that on and so can you.

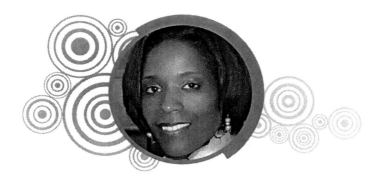

Melody McClellan, CHHC, AADP

Melody McClellan is the founder of Unwrap You. She is a graduate of Southern Illinois University at Edwardsville and majored in business administration with an emphasis in marketing. Also, she is an award winning pharmaceutical representative (fourteen years) specializing in diabetes, cholesterol, obesity, and weight management.

As a certified health coach, she personalizes workshops, speaking engagements, corporate wellness, and group programs on various topics dealing with health. Her goal is to educate and improve the outcome of women and girls by altering lifestyles and making sustainable changes that will produce real and lasting results.

She resides in O'Fallon, Illinois, with her husband of nineteen years and two teenage sons.

www.unwrapyou.com

✉ **coachmelody@unwrapyou.com**

f **Unwrap you with Coach Melody**

in **Melody McClellan**

CHAPTER 26

YOUR DREAMS ARE POSSIBLE

By Melody McClellan, CHHC, AADP

It all started for me when I was born to a teenage mother and grew up in the inner city of Los Angeles. I knew at a very young age I wanted to change my future by first attending and graduating from a four-year university, then getting married before having any children and raising them in a two-parent home. This was very important to me because of the struggles I witnessed with my mother. She was our sole provider, with no support, and worked so hard to provide for me and my brother. As a result, I understood the importance of waiting and making sure I could care for my family properly. This meant early on I would prefer to share this life-changing experience with a spouse. There were others that helped shape my character. My grandmother, aunts, uncles, and mentors were encouraging me along the way to be my best.

I have always been a talker, and passionate about selling. Family knew early on I had a future that would include marketing and sales. My first working experience was at the age of twelve, selling subscriptions for the *Oakland Tribune*. I actually won my first sales contest with the most subscriptions sold for the month. The manager stated, "Melody is a natural-born salesperson"—something my mother reminds me of when we reflect on my past. Take time to explore those natural gifts and talents we all have. It is a matter of recognizing then refining them.

I became aware of the benefits of health and wellness when I was eighteen years old. After researching healthier food options and the benefits of exercising, I knew it was time to reshape my body. Along with this idea came a complete overhaul of all the foods I had been fed growing up. I eliminated many food items and incorporated new habits like lean meats, baked foods, fruits and raw veggies. I even became a vegetarian. This lifestyle had become very important to me, helping me to develop the habits needed to incur life-changing results. Soon after, I had a knee injury. I was derailed but determined not to allow this injury to set me back. I immediately formulated a plan to stay consistent, accountable, and continue to maintain the best body. By incorporating exercise and healthier habits and decreasing my weight, I increased energy, which was something I had become accustomed to and had no plans of stopping.

A large part of my growth was leaving Los Angeles at twenty years of age and moving to Illinois to attend college. Of course, it was my choice to attend a four-year university but two thousand miles was far from home. I remember wanting to quit but my mother encouraged me to finish out the year. I am glad she did because eventually I adapted to my surroundings and succeeded by graduating four years later with a degree in business administration with an emphasis in marketing.

I met my husband as a student in college. We have been together for nineteen years, and this relationship has been a work in progress. Taking proper time to love, nurture, and respect our commitment takes work because we are still individuals. We have been through a lot since college, starting with raising children, establishing careers, as well as several moves, which helped us grow as a couple. Our relationship has lasted because we share responsibilities, listen to one another, and work together and it attributes to us staying together. Here are a few tips to keep a healthy marriage while working, having kids, and managing a home:

- GOD-centered prayer
- Church home – couples classes
- Always communicate
- Date each other – intimacy
- Compromise and don't feel like you have to win

I have seen so many marriages end in the past ten years. You have to stay committed. There will be trials, periods of change, new directions, new opportunities, but stay focused on your vows. Continue to communicate and never go to bed angry. Life is too short, with no time to waste your precious moments on trivial things.

After graduating college, I pursued a career in pharmaceutical sales. As a sales professional in the medical field, I had to balance family, career, and social activities. The pharmaceutical industry is very selective with intense training. People refer to it as going back to mini-medical school because of the intense training. There is a comprehensive understanding of the disease state, testing of knowledge, learning the competition, and being proficient to sell the medication. Another huge accomplishment!

In my optimistic mind, I imagined managing it all would be easy. I would start with my relationship, kids, work, social life and it would be perfect. Reality quickly set in, and I realized I would need to find balance and prioritize life events by creating a schedule, concluding everything did not have to be perfect or immaculate at all times. No need to create a stressful environment at home, so I changed my thought process and approach. This helped me maintain my sanity. My motto: "If it can't get done today, there is always tomorrow."

Taking care of our two sons and making sure they had what was needed to get them to the next level in life has been our priority. Even though I have had a demanding career, I missed very few games, parent-teacher conferences, meetings, and activities.

When raising children, we are not perfect or may not have all the answers but we make sure we do our very best.

TIPS:

- Do everything in LOVE
- Make quality time (enjoy events)
- Be present when together (no electronics)
- Sit and eat at least one meal together (share your day)

Having quality time and supporting my kids has been very important to me.

Life is constantly changing. The majority of my adult life has been as a wife and mother then the SHIFT. I absolutely love my family and what has been accomplished thus far but noticed a change taking place. For years, I have been the go to person with family and friends asking *what should I eat, how much should I eat,* and *can you help*?

In 2013, I took my years of medical experience specializing in diabetes, cholesterol, weight management, and obesity and started my year-long certification in nutrition school to become a health coach, which was a complement to my experience and background. This idea had been brewing for eight years and I finally stepped out on faith to pursue my passion of helping women accomplish their goals in health and wellness. I successfully completed the program and received my health coaching certification. During the same year, I started my business, Unwrap You. I create and facilitate health and wellness programs that help women reveal the happy, healthy person inside.

You know the saying, "Do what you are passionate about or what you would do for free"? Exactly what I was seeking to pursue and finally accomplished.

There are misconceptions with physical activity and nutrition—like *eat less* and *lose weight*, but this is not always the answer. If it was that, easy there would not be a rapid rise in obesity. It is important to make sure you are in balance with all three aspects: mind, body, and spirit.

"Everybody is beautiful," but if you don't like something, change it.

Some keys factors:

- Eat to nourish the body
- Smaller portions = small plate
- Drink water to hydrate your body
- Physical activity – do what you enjoy – stay consistent
- Self-care- massage- quiet time

The goal is to become the best YOU, so make sure you are in balance. Small things can get you off course. It is important to have the right state of mind, body, and spirit to assure long-term success.

There is not a quick fix to lifestyle change, but the journey is ongoing to create the best you. It is so important to walk in your purpose by staying determined and focused. You can achieve the goals if you set them. Make sure you have the correct strategies and techniques in place to succeed. This is the time to sit back and access your choices, direction, and then redirect if needed.

Phrase I live by:

> "Nothing will work unless you do."
>
> ~ Maya Angelou

Looking back on my life, I did not have it all. It was not perfect but it was my life. Being determined as a young girl to make positive changes and remain focused on not being a statistic, I was able to overcome so many obstacles and change my outcome. With that, I have stayed married, have wonderful family, a college education, a successful career, and am starting a new business. I have accomplished my goals and so can you.

Remember, how you start is not how it ends because you get to reshape and tell your own story. Dream it! Believe it! Achieve it!

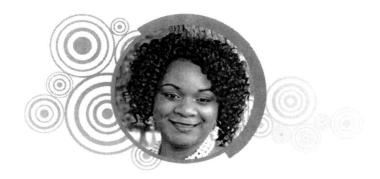

N'kia Jones Campbell, EdS

I am N'kia Jones Campbell—a Christian, a wife, an educator, a mother, a daughter, a sister, a doctoral student, a niece, a friend, and a ball of energy, to say the least. I have served as an educator for over sixteen years, in various capacities: teacher, assistant principal, principal, and currently a director of academic initiatives, and one day, a district superintendent. Throughout all of my interactions, I find myself speaking from life experiences. Instead of lessons that I have taught, I speak candidly of the lessons that I have learned throughout my career path.

✉ **nkia.campbell@gmail.com**
❶ **facebook.com/nkia.campbell**
🐦 **twitter.com/NkiaCampbell**

CHAPTER 27

THE TRUE LESSONS TO CAREER HAPPINESS

By N'kia Jones Campbell, EdS

Growing up as a little girl on a remote island off the coast of South Carolina brought about many fascinating experiences! Both parents worked in the public school system. I remember playing in my father's classroom and my mother always telling me that I could do all things through Christ. I knew early on that teaching was going to be my career path!

At age seven, I would always play the role of the teacher. My younger brother, childhood friends, pets, and stuffed animals were always my students. And yes, I differentiated instruction; I conferenced with my students and I gave homework! But it was three years later that my decision to become a teacher was cemented.

I met my fifth grade teacher. She was different from all my other teachers. She walked differently, she dressed differently, and she expected something different: "THE BEST!" It was love at first sight! Every day, she would come dressed in a two-piece business suit with three-inch high heel shoes. She would have on just the right amount of makeup; her hair was always done to perfection. She would enter the room like she was president of the United States. She would reach into her business bag and pull out a ripe banana. She would slowly peel the banana back, eat it, and begin the day with…"Class, you are here to learn. You need to get your education, because it doesn't come cheap. You must learn to love to read, because this is the ONLY way that you will succeed." This was a mantra! Her expectations were out of the roof. She treated us like young adults, not ten-year-old children.

As I matriculated through high school, I always kept my fifth grade experience in the forefront of every decision I made. My senior year of high school, I registered for the teacher cadet program. After high school graduation, I attended Winthrop University in Rock Hill, South Carolina—one of the best teaching colleges in the southeast. At Winthrop, I majored in elementary education. I knew without a shadow of a doubt, I wanted to emulate my fifth grade teacher. I also knew that I wanted to return to my community to give back.

In May of 1998, I graduated with a bachelor's of science degree. I interviewed for a teaching position in my hometown and was offered a fourth grade position. I was happy that I was now employed; however, I was disappointed that I was not teaching fifth grade. At the end of my first year of teaching, I enrolled in a graduate program in Charleston, South Carolina. Two years later, I graduated with a master's degree in educational leadership and I was teaching fifth grade. Life was GREAT! What else could I ask for? I was twenty-five years old, and I was at my happiest in my life..

That summer, I was offered an assistant principal position at a feeder middle school. I really LOVED the classroom, and I LOVED my students. I knew that this position would give me the platform that I could use to help so many more students. I accepted the position and became the youngest administrator in the district. More ironically, I was charged with supervising teachers whose teaching experience exceeded my young age. In order to set myself up for success, I knew early on that my approach to instructional leadership was going to be collaborative in nature. To me, having a shared vision was important.

One of the first lessons I learned in this leadership role was the importance of building relationships. Every opportunity I had, I made sure that I was accessible to teachers and I took a personal interest in them. With this established philosophy, I knew that this was the foundation for building a successful school environment.

In 2004, I was awarded a Fulbright scholarship to teach in Ghana, West Africa, for eight weeks. I knew this was going to be an opportunity of a lifetime. This was my first time traveling out of the country, let alone staying out of the United States. I would be gone for two months. I was so excited at first, but the closer I got to the date of departure, the fear of the unknown started to sink in. I kept telling myself negative things. I felt like the only way to escape this negative energy was to stick to the status quo and not go.

But a lovely friend said to me, "N'kia, you have to go! You will never forgive yourself if you don't. As a black woman, you owe it to your ancestors to return to the motherland. Not many people get this opportunity." That summer, I participated in the Charleston Southern University-Ghana West Africa Teaching and Learning Experience. For eight weeks, I lived in Ghana, West Africa. I taught village children from various ages. I ate, slept, and played in the village. I met kings and queens, but most of all, I learned so much about myself.

One year after returning from Ghana, I got married to my soul mate. We'd dated off and on for four years. I knew the moment I saw him, he was special and he was the one. We were engaged for a few months before I flew to Ghana. My experiences in Ghana solidified my love for him. Everywhere we went in the West African country, we saw symbols of love and unity that reminded me of our relationship. I could not imagine myself without him. He was my king!

Being married taught me how to support and care for someone else. Together, I knew we could conquer the world. For seven years, I climbed the professional ladder as a single woman. The decisions I made affected me and my future only. As a wife, I had to factor my husband's dreams and aspirations into the equation, and find ways that we both could support each other.

At the age of thirty, I was named principal of an elementary school. Again, I was the youngest principal in the district. In the first year as principal, the school received a state award, the Palmetto Silver Award, for improving student achievement. As a school, we did a tremendous amount to impact student achievement. We made gains but not the gains that we had hoped to see. Like the cliché that we are all too familiar with, *it takes time to see true results*. Unfortunately, I had sacrificed almost everything to be the successful principal that everyone expected me to be.

I sacrificed my marriage, friendships, my health, and so much more to improve test scores! Was it worth everything that I sacrificed for the first year as principal? I had a husband who got injured in the Iraq War that needed my support. The role of a principal seemed to be more about putting out fires than addressing the true needs of the students. For the first time in my life, I felt unsuccessful. I felt like I was not getting the return on my investment. I wanted something more. I wanted to be a mother.

My husband and I wanted to start a family. We tried for three years to have a child, but unfortunately, we struggled. We had a miscarriage and were later diagnosed with infertility. Having a baby seemed impossible. I had given up. I questioned God. Why was he not answering our prayer? Why was everyone else having children? It seemed so unfair. Up to that point, everything I had accomplished, I *wanted* to accomplish. I realized that having a baby was not up to me, but up to God. Our inability to have a child reinforced my feeling of failure. In August of 2010, we learned that I was pregnant. Nine months later, God blessed us with a healthy baby girl. We named her Naomi Rose.

I was a new mother. Out of all my experiences in the school system, the role of a mother was quite challenging to say the least, but it has also been the most rewarding. It was the first year of Naomi's life, I learned about true sacrifice. I found myself going without so that she could have.

Yet my roles switched again—I was no longer the teacher or the principal but the student. My new learning target was being able to care about the happiness of another person without any thought for what I might get for myself. It did not matter what position I held, it was the small things that counted most.

Ironically enough, my little one was now the teacher. She was teaching me life lessons on commitment, giving, patience, and happiness, but the most valuable lesson that Naomi was teaching me was the lesson of unconditional LOVE. Through all of my life experiences, I realized that these experiences were prerequisites for the next chapter of my life.

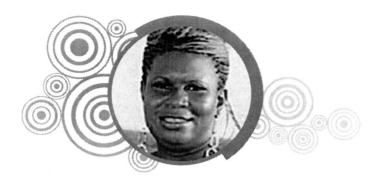

Terry Dais-Pasley

When you hear TDP Consulting, you recognize not only the "brand" but the CEO— Founder Terry Dais-Pasley: wife, mother, grandmother, entrepreneur, business owner, and now author. As a business consultant, Terry works with clients to increase awareness about their products and services. She and her team accomplish this through advertising, consulting, marketing, networking, and promotions. Originally from Charleston, SC, Terry has lived in Indianapolis and Florida. She returned to her roots and is building one of the premier marketing agencies in the Low Country area, and across the globe. Terry enjoys this venture with her husband John, daughters Ashley, A'Kahla, and Julana, and grandson A'Kheal.

www.tdpconsulting.net

✉ **terry@tdpconsulting.net**

f **facebook.com/TDPCONSULTN**

◉ **instgram.com/TDPCONSULTN**

℗ **pinterest.com/consulttdp/**

✆ **twitter.com/TDPCONSULTN**

CHAPTER 28

ENTREPRENEURSHIP AS A CAREER!

By Terry Dais-Pasley

The all-so familiar announcements of corporate downsizing and company layoffs. I remember the cold winter Friday like it was yesterday. My supervisor John called a mandatory meeting to discuss the immediate departmental changes. My first thought was we would be getting promoted. The entire department had been working diligently on this project. In fact, most of us were working sixteen-hour days. You would think the insurance industry was a stable profession for agents. Four state licenses, several certifications, and eight years later, I found myself fretting every day for my job. The uncertainties of not knowing when I would receive my next paycheck didn't sit well with me.

My frequent self-evaluations always lead me to step out on faith and seek new opportunities. This time was no different. Three years prior, I decided that I needed to earn more money to help take care of my family. I began sending my resume out to companies in Florida, North Carolina, and Virginia. Little did I know, the response would come so quick. In forty-eight hours, I was offered a position with a large insurance agency. The job was three and a half hours away and started in ten days. I had always done well in the industry. This new venture would give me the start I needed into project management! In fact, the company was contracted to work with the insurance commission of the state of Florida. This was certain to be the "big break" I was looking for.

My family, on the other hand, didn't see the need to relocate. They loved Charleston and didn't want to leave their comfort zone. I was persistent about making this change and pursuing a new opportunity. With the majority of my support system against my decision, I contacted a friend in Jacksonville and I was on my way. I arrived on Monday—Labor Day—and my job started the very next day. New city, new job, and time to find a new place to live. My first day of training went well. You know the excitement of learning new systems, software programs, and meeting new coworkers. It all seemed to be well worth the move for the first two and a half years.

The water cooler and break room chatter began. Treece asked, "Has anyone heard that our project is ending?" "Did anyone see an article in the Sunday newspaper bashing the decision of the insurance commission to do this project?" I don't watch TV much, and barely read the newspaper, so I didn't have a response. I was always working. I began to look and listen for signs at work. A few weeks went by, and there was a decline in our workload and a few changes in responsibility. Surely there was something unusual happening. The thoughts running through my head began to consume me. I knew I didn't relocate here to lose my job. I'm well aware that certain things are only for a season, and maybe this season was over. What would I do now? I thought I had my career all figured out. I truly enjoyed working at the insurance company, but the entrepreneur in me was always planning a business.

In the midst of everything at work, I met Treece. Her family was originally from Charleston but relocated to Jacksonville when she was young. She had spent some years in Atlanta and decided to move back to Jax, make some money, and start her business. The talk of our job ending encouraged us to start a business. Treece sold human hair extensions, and my daughter Julana was a licensed cosmetologist. I thought this would be great—we could open a salon and give my daughter a reason to move to Jacksonville. We solidfied our business plans, and opened the WOW Salon JAX. This was an amazing hair and nail salon located on the Southside of Jacksonville, Florida. we began hiring professional hair stylists, along with nail technicians. I definitely wanted my daughter to be included, but after careful consideration she decided not to relocate. While I enjoyed being a Co-Owner of the Salon, the hair industry wasn't my passion. It was time to review, revise and revamp my plans.

When I arrived to work on Monday morning, I was advised that there was a department meeting scheduled for that afternoon. My supervisor started the meeting on a positive note. We were told that if we heard anything on the news or read anything in the newspapers, to take it with a grain of salt. The project was here to stay and no one would be losing their jobs. The meeting definitely increased the morale of the department, but I wasn't convinced. I began to meditate and spent numerous hours in prayer. I would go to bed reading my Bible and woke up doing the same thing. My daily prayer was: *Lord, please bless me with my own business. I don't ever want to be in a situation where I'm not in control of my destiny or my salary.* In subtle ways, the Lord began to answer my prayer. I could feel it—a change was coming.

Two months later, a church sister contacted me. She wanted to know if I would help her market and promote her book. Advertising, marketing, promotions, and public speaking are a few areas of my expertise. I was excited about the opportunity and the potential of working with other authors. My creative juices began to flow and I immediately started working on her campaign. I had done this type of project on many occasions but for free. This time I would be doing it for a client. I began to contemplate what to charge her for my services. I spent a lot of time on social media. A friend from Charleston was always talking about her new business. I decided to contact her for some advice. She was excited for me but didn't want to give me any advice on pricing. She referred me to her business coach. I contacted her and it was like we had known each other for twenty years. She began to question me about my background and current and future goals. Immediately, she said, "This sounds like a business that you would be good at. You already have lots of experience. " The lights went on and I started TDP Public Relations Agency in Jacksonville.

Six months later, we received notification that our project was ending. The holidays were coming, and I was heading to Charleston to be with my family. Now, the dilemma began. Stay in Jacksonville and look for another job, or move back home and build this business? It was the day before Thanksgiving, and I hit the road, excited to see family and friends but contemplating my big decision. My friend encouraged me to read *The Dream Killer*. It was as though this book took over my life. The author was speaking directly to me. I didn't speak during the entire drive home. We reached the *Welcome to South Carolina* sign, and I reached my decision. No longer would I just be an employee with entrepreneurial tendencies, but I would begin my career as an entrepreneur!

I told my coach of my decision and I began to execute my formal business training. Just like the character in *The Dream Killer*, my family members began their mission to kill my dreams. I have always been a strong-willed woman and now was no different. The "ram" in me was determined to only allow one man to dictate my future. I decided to truly build a personal relationship with God. I began attending noon day prayer service, praying more, reading more, and studying the word of God! Every day I prayed for my business. I worked countless hours, even when I only had one client. You see, being an entrepreneur isn't an easy task. If it was, everyone would be doing it. I stood on the word of God's grace and mercy. In time, he began to show me "favor" over my business. No more seeking a career. My God provided me a career as an entrepreneur when he made me. The unique gifts and talents that he has only blessed Terry Dais-Pasley with have awarded me the opportunity to start my business. TDP Consulting is building and growing by leaps and bounds! Successful people do what unsuccessful people aren't willing to do. "Build Your Business!"

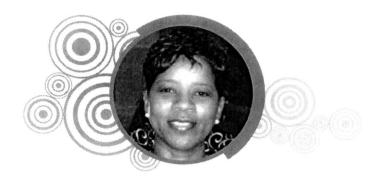

Mary Evelyn Caudle

Elected as Mayor of the Town of Triana in 2008, Mary E. Caudle has presided over some dramatic transformations in the town's history. In 1996, she founded ASSIST Practice Management Services, LLC, after sixteen years in the medical field. Mary is the proud mother of three children; LaToya, Ian, and Brandon, and grandmother of four; Briana, Jalen, Jada and Brandon J. Mary serves on the board of directors of Top of Alabama Regional Council of Governments, Metropolitan Planning Organization for Huntsville/ Madison Counties, and Community Action Partnership for Madison and Limestone Counties, and was president of the North Alabama Mayors Association in 2013-2014.

CHAPTER 29

LEANING FORWARD

By Mary Evelyn Caudle

Born to a rural farmer and housewife, into a family of ten children, my life has always been engulfed by role models who were a daily inspiration and an example of sacrifice that meets triumph—my story would be no different. My legacy would start earlier than expected but would never be the end of the story. At the age of sixteen, I gave birth to my first child and had to immediately focus on a new first goal for life. Graduating from high school was essential to meet the career goals that I had envisioned. After graduating from high school in 1977 and beginning my first year of college, I suffered another small regroup of plans as I gave birth to my second child. Being a mother included working multiple jobs and enduring late nights and early mornings as I struggled to keep up with the demands of being a mother and employee.

In 1982, I began my first career move that would be the beginning of my continuous focus to play a vital role in providing of medical services to people who are uninsured or underinsured. As a receptionist with a Federal Qualified Healthcare Center (FQHC), I engaged in an early opportunity to lean toward my future goals. This position provided an introduction and experience in the medical services field that would be a stepping stone for me and my future.

At the age of twenty-one, I would take a big step forward with no looking back. I built my first home for my children and married two years later in 1983. Setting my sites on entrepreneurship, I started early and bought a small trailer that I kept on my property and began my own business as a seamstress. I was determined, by any means necessary, to provide for my children while having a business mindset. Two years later, I gave birth to my third child. However, the marriage ended in 1987 and I found myself with three children, still leaning forward—searching and expecting a better future in my career.

After eight years of developing skills necessary for corporate level management in medical services, I embarked upon a new position that was one more step up the ladder to reaching my ultimate goal of owning my own business. As director of financial services for a local company, I knew that seeking small opportunities were necessary to create great moves in my career. Always pressing forward, I found myself serving as the liaison between facilities and corporate accounting. While working diligently in the position for six years assisting the company in gaining financial stability, my desire to continue to serve those that are uninsured or underinsured led the way to my return to the company that was my first job. This next step on the ladder was as a director of revenue management services. For the next nine years, I would be responsible for overall corporate accounts and collaboration with the management team to develop and refine corporate level goals. The continuous learning along the way and drive to lead facilities to another level was a constant focus for me. It was evident for me that I had empowered myself with the tools to take a step forward by starting my own consulting business. For the next few years, I would prepare mentally and financially for this gigantic step in my life.

As a result of inquiries from similar medical facilities to the one that I was currently working, I developed a realization that my qualifications could be marketable. Seeing a need for these services led me to initiate my own consultant services that I would manage from my home. After an introduction to twenty-five FQHC facilities with a simple letter outlining my available consultant services, my path was lit by contact from three facilities—my business was launched.

For the next two years, I would provide medical consultation in the areas of accounts receivable management, revenue management, and billing/collecting services. As I continued to focus on the future of the business and family, I saved all profits in an effort to reach my goal of building and owning my very own office space. In February

2006, ASSIST Practice Management had a home! Four months later, I resigned my full-time job and pressed forward full time with my business.

As my business began to thrive, I shifted my focus on how I could assist the community in which I resided and where my business was located. My community is extra special due to the fact that it is also home to where my grandparents, parents, myself, and children were born, raised, and continue to reside. This encouraged me to run and be successfully elected as part of the Town of Triana council. Serving four years in this position was only the beginning of my political career. During this time, I realized the potential of the town and I knew I could make a difference. Also, I felt that I could play a vital role in the process of change. This encouraged me to prepare for my desired goal to become mayor of the Town of Triana. In 2008, I was elected mayor. Embarking in this new responsibility, my goal was to grow the community and push forward for change! My commitment to ensuring safety for all citizens led me to improve the emergency services. In an effort to increase the quality of life for the citizens, I worked tirelessly on securing grants that assisted in the revitalizing of the town park, rebuilding the town public library, and assisting elderly with home repairs. While continuing to work with landowners and developers, the town gained two new subdivisions that had the potential to bring one thousand new citizens to the community. During my tenure, the largest improvement that resulted was diversity — while still preserving the history of the town.

I still continued to grow my personal business while working as mayor of the Town of Triana. Now serving my second term, the position has empowered me with the opportunity to represent not only my community but other communities while serving on several elected board positions. For the 2012-2013 fiscal year, I served as vice president; and for 2013-2014, president of the North Alabama Mayors Association. I also serve on the board of directors for the Community Action Agency where local mayors, other governmental agencies, and citizens collaborate regarding situations within their community in an effort to improve their own communities. Since 2009, I've played a vital role as part of the Top of Alabama Regional Council of Governments (TARCOG) board of directors. In correlation with the goals of my town, I worked with the board to obtain funding that will improve the quality of life for all citizens of North Alabama.

In January 2012, my career would take another lean forward as ASSIST received a client that would change the path of my career. Beginning as a consultant, I would make an impact on the company's accounts receivables and special projects, thus leading to a company financial recovery that resulted in the offer of a contract position within the company. This position allowed me to serve as corporate director of accounts receivable/special projects, which provides services through-out the Unites States.

No amount of adversities would stop me from reaching goals and achieving success in several areas of my career. It's never too late to reach set goals. As I proudly support my three children, who have all earned college degrees, I know that I have one more goal to reach—to obtain my own BS college degree.

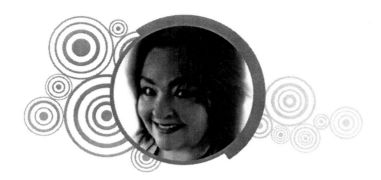

Carla Wynn Hall

Carla Wynn Hall is a passionate writer who brilliantly creates words that empower and inspire. As a mother of three sons, she knows the power of persistence and the grace of being a mom.

Currently Carla Wynn Hall is the CEO/Founder of Sacred Heart Woman, a branding solution for the "WooPreneur" or woman who wants a website to totally and fully connect with her inner core and personality classification. She claims that women must have a branding campaign that creates happiness.

www.empoweredwomenofsocialmedia.com

facebook.com/empoweredwomenofsocialmedia

twitter.com/carlawynnhall

linkedin.com/in/carlawynnhall

CHAPTER 30

TAP AWAY DISEASE AND PHYSICAL ILLNESS

By Carla Wynn Hall

My story began as many too, in the dark catacombs of my mind where past memories had taken residence and set out on a mission to destroy me from the inside out. It is my full belief that our thoughts and choices in life, whether positive or negative, create physical manifestations in our bodies. My name is Carla Wynn Hall and I would like to tell you my story of how I learned how to use a process called memory transmutation to shift my life, heal my body and illuminate my spirit.

In the beginning of my story to purposeful health and well-being, I want to tell you just a little about how my mental and emotional state of mind developed over the course of my lifetime and how the emotional issues I had inherited through DNA from my lineage. I was born the daughter of a factory worker and a homemaker. My mother is and always has been beautiful with amazing skin, black hair (now gray) and light blue eyes. My father is ½ Cherokee Indian and has black (now gray) hair with deep brown eyes. My parents consistently practiced eating habits akin of poverty, lack and fear. By this I mean a diet full of floury, starchy foods that have nearly no nutritional value.

Often I would arrive home from school and supper would already be on the table. There would be biscuits, gravy and friend deer meet. We were made to eat all of our food without fail or we were in serious trouble. We, meaning myself and my two younger sisters. When we are children we have no choice but to follow the guidelines of our parents. We learn as small children to eat with almost every emotion. With sadness our moms would make cookies or cake. With birthdays more cake and even at church events we were exposed to tables upon tables of casseroles and desserts.

How does emotional eating as a child and using our conscious thoughts to become more mindful of the importance of staying healthy form an educational pathway to greater overall well-being? In my humble opinion there is no separation in our mind, body or spirit. When one is inflicted such as with a poverty mindset, the other is affected and responds in kind. This manifestation can appear as diabetes, obesity and even yeast infections.

My childhood had a direct impact on my adult hood and I did develop Type II Diabetes that first appeared in my 2nd and 3rd pregnancy requiring me to inject insulin into my leg or arm daily. Looking back at my childhood I was different than my sisters. I had a different metabolism. I gained weight easy and they stayed lean. My family was inflicted with a poverty mindset. There is no doubt that the food choices my mother made for her children, resulted in the manifestation of eating diseases.

Fast forward to 2014, the year of the writing of this "OhMazing" book. Today I am aware of the true fact that our emotions have a direct impact on our physical health. In 2010 I started using a mind/body/ spirit practice called EFT Tapping. Emotional Freedom Technique is a method to release emotions that are toxic in nature. It requires a simply physical action of tapping certain body points with your hand to activate part of our system called "Meridians". Meridians are energy centers in our bodies that are found from head to toe.

When I first started tapping, I wanted to release the emotions that were causing my blood sugar to stay high. I was sick and I didn't want to take medication for this disorder. I have always been very much against synthetic medications. To truly embrace EFT one must believe in the power of the unseen forces around us. To truly embrace 100% health, we must know that our bodies are capable of changing if we believe they can change.

Emotional Freedom Technique helps you release trapped energy that has kept you stuck for so long. It is a process that combines the physical act of tapping with your fingertips, with a process of affirmations and celebration. Affirmations are sets of instructions you start to say and repeat them over and over. The result is that you begin to change your "belief pathway" and literally reprogram your DNA. I would like to give you a simple EFT sequence to use to connect mind, spirit and body in a process that will help shift your body and mind.

5 EFT Affirmations to do daily for 21 days with the intention of releasing emotions that are associated with eating diseases.

Keep note of these affirmations for future use. Using your first three fingers on either hand start by tapping your opposite hand just below your pinky finger on the fleshy part of your hand called the "Karate Chop Point". Start with deep breathing and conviction, then say these affirmations out loud.

1. **My body mind and soul are in perfect harmony.**
2. **All of my drainage pathways are always clear.**
3. **The happier I am the better I feel.**
4. **I love, accept and forgive myself totally.**
5. **My body functions at 100% every single day.**

I realized once I started to say these things to myself, some part of me would rise up as if to pose an invisible argument. The first step in using your spirit and mind to heal your body is to know that you have old beliefs that may hold you back from being healthy. When you can recognize these emotions and release the blocks, you will be free. Until then you just choose to "Fake it" until you "Make it" by using these affirmations with a soulful intention that your health will improve if you say so.

My journey of tapping started with my commitment to do affirmations for 21 days. When I first started, my ego, the voice in my head, kept saying that I needed to go to the doctor. My soul, however, sought deeply to heal this disease by dealing with the emotional energy that was keeping diabetes hanging around. On day one, I felt a unique energy surging through me. The more I said the affirmations, the more I believed them.

The affirmations I said were focused on Type II Diabetes and Panic Attacks. An example of an affirmation I did for Type II Diabetes was "I am free of diabetes and have always been free of diabetes as long as I can remember" and "I love my pancreas because it keeps my insulin flowing". For panic attacks I would do the same thing but include "I am 100% safe in this present moment and I am at peace". We have heard these affirmations from great leaders such as Louis Hay author of "You can heal your Life"; and from movies such as The Secret (Rhonda Byrn). Listen to them and listen to me as I guide you gently into the world of magical transformation.

After 7 days of tapping I had lost 30 pounds and was drinking 100 ounces of water a day. Not only that but my eyes brightened and my step was pepped. I knew something was working so I decided to increase the vibration of my affirmations adding a WOO HOO to the end of each one and drinking water between tapping affirmations. Someone had told me that water was the source of spirit in our bodies and I listened. After day 21 I checked my glucose and it was 100, the lowest it had been in 3 years.

In closing let me say that being healthy is the key to your longevity and the health and welfare of your children and grandchildren. Today I have three grandchildren ages 9, 2 and (not yet born). To show them the power of self-healing through creating health mind habits, is my passion.

I am the author of The Paradigm Success Codes for Life: In the Catacombs of the Subconscious. My passion is in showing women the magic and power that reveals itself to them if they will only take the journey. Remember the longest road or the shortest path begins with a single step. Understanding that your mind can cause illness in your body, and when you release emotions that exists only to hold your body back, you are starting a new path toward true wellness.

Allow your heart to forgive anyone for any reason. Visualize your body as you want it to be, perfect in every say. Repeat your affirmations every day. Celebrate your success. Today is the only day you have so live it with honor and bliss. Be well and have an amazing life.

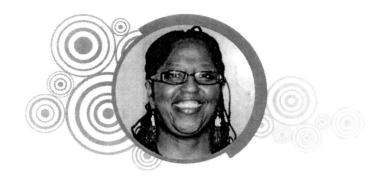

Joyce Swinson

Joyce Swinson is a financial service professional, specializing in increasing financial literacy for women, families, and young professionals. Providing quality financial strategies and offering insurance, financial products and services, and employee benefits services to businesses and individuals, Joyce became an agent with New York Life Insurance Company after even years in the business development industry and over twenty years as a mental health therapist. Joyce is a native Washingtonian and has traveled extensively throughout the US, Ghana, and Mexico teaching financial literacy and business development. She resides in the DC area with her husband of twenty-eight years and their two children.

Joyce Swinson can be reached at:

✉ **wealthdiva32@gmail.com**

f **facebook.com/joyce.swinson32**

CHAPTER 31

FINANCIAL WELLNESS

By Joyce Swinson

"...Thus saith the Lord, thy Redeemer, the Holy One of Israel; I am the Lord thy God which teacheth thee to profit..." Isaiah 48:17

The first thing I embraced in order to have a healthy financial lifestyle is that we live in a world of abundance. Money is plentiful—not scarce, and resources abound. When I was young and didn't know this principle and didn't have enough money, I used to pay bills by colors, similar to the paint-by-numbers pictures of old! If the bill came in a colored envelop or the window was colored, it meant that the utility had a cutoff date inside. I would muster up all the money I could to pay that bill and the others would have to wait to get paid when their color came up next! This brings us to our first key of financial wellness: Know that you are blessed. God wants us to live an abundant life and has given us the power to get wealth! (Duet 8:18) Our gifts, our talents, our jobs, and our skills all are sources of potential income or power for us to receive this wealth.

We must put God first in all we do—in prayer and communication (Matthew 6:33), in our thoughts and our actions (Prov. 3:6), and of course in our finances (Lev. 23:10). We are commanded to bring our tithe into the store house (Mal. 3:10). Therefore, all messages that I teach always begin with putting our finances in the correct order so that we can line up with the word of God. To set aside a tenth of all of our income, regardless of which resource it is spun from, is first on our list of steps to financial wellness. Many cultures and religions acknowledge giving first to God as foundational.

Once we have paid our tithe, then we invest in ourselves, or as some sources say, "Pay yourself." Even fruit has enough sense to produce seed to be planted so it can reproduce and make more fruit—so must we by investing in ourselves a portion of each increase. We can decide on a specific amount or a certain percentage of our incoming monies. The purpose of this money is for our future use and eventually will require more sophisticated ways of growth (return) other than a savings account that pays very little interest.

With the remainder of the monies from our income or business ventures, we then develop a financial plan, a spending plan—a budget if you will! Here is where you gather all of your bills, debts, assets, and financial accounts so you can sort and see where you stand. And then map out a strategic plan to where you want to go. This exercise will take some searching to find each account, and you will need to forecast down the line to see what bills or payments are on the horizon, like the purchase of a home, college for the children, to start a business, to travel the world. I remember when I was drowning in debt and couldn't see my way out because I didn't have any idea how much I owed and to whom I owed. My finances were out of control. I decided to take the bull by the horns and gathered all of my bills, utilities, and statements. I laid all of them on the sofa and I sat in a chair in front of them to conduct a business meeting! "I have called you all together today to inform you that I am taking control of my financial future and to announce to most of you bills that you are no longer a welcomed part of my life. You will be exiting soon—and very soon. Today, I am setting in motion a plan to evict you out of my life," I proudly announced. "And to you bank accounts and investment statements, and all of you other assets that make my money multiply, to you I proclaim, you will be growing quite rapidly!"

With the help of a wonderful, practical financial advisor, we developed a strategic plan to get us out of debt and to improve our credit score. We developed a strategic savings plan that encompassed two different saving goals 1) Long-term (3-6 months of expenses in case our job situation changed suddenly) and retirement 2) Short-term (car maintenance, vacations, shoes—didn't think I'd leave those to chance)! I read every book I could find on getting out of debt and saving and building generational wealth.

Once my goals were set and this plan was developed, the best part of my journey was to automate everything. At first, I was leery of doing so much of my personal financial business online but it was the best strategy ever! It is easier now more than ever before in our history to automatically save money, invest money, pay bills, and buy things that we need online with a click of a mouse! Our paychecks are deposited directly into our bank accounts and we can determine where the money goes from there. Our bills get paid on time, which helps our credit score. Our savings grow exponentially when we automatically put our money in accounts that we don't have easy access to before we've even had a chance to miss it. When we become more conscious in our spending and saving, we take out the middlemen of waste and careless spending.

Now that we have God first, invested in ourselves secondly, and developed and automated a strategic financial spending and savings plan, it's time for us to live out our lives of financial wellness through our giving! Yes, I said giving.

When we take the stress and strain out of our lives by organizing and clearing away the handcuffs of debt and overextending ourselves, we can see just how much this frees us up to focus outward to others. We can bless others on purpose and intentionally. We can give more value to our family, friends, and society. Be a giver of your time, your talent, and your treasure. Don't forget to bless people with your words of praise and encouragement, too. When I decided to put my financial house in order and experienced the freedom of being debt-free and financially stable, I could then reach out to others and help them find the same thing. And this encouragement soon led to the fulfillment of the call on my life to help others live an abundant life in financial wellness!

- I now teach financial literacy to children through games, activities, and money camps so they become financially responsible children that grow up to be financially responsible adults.
- I now help college students plan for their future income and set in places financial systems to handle the big j-o-b that comes after graduate.

- I now help young families who were in the same crazy money situations (like too much credit card debt and student loan debt and no savings and too much private school tuition) that my husband and I were in twenty-five years ago (we've been married twenty-eight years this year, to God be the glory!) I can share with them what I know now that I didn't know twenty-eight years ago and wish somebody would have shared with me, i.e. protect your family with life insurance (someone may get sick and not be able to get it when they get older, or you might want to start a business later on in life and you can use some of the money in your life insurance policy to help fund your start up); or if you just put $25 aside each payday, it will add up before you know it. Even though you may not be able to conceive it now, the children will grow up and leave your house and you will need money to go to the beach without them to celebrate "their independence!"

- I now help people who didn't have anyone to say those things to them or those who heard and didn't believe it then and now need to "catch up" because retirement is quickly coming into view. We've been able to create tax-free buckets of income that will help them in those retirement years.

- I now have time to read postcards from all over the world and see pictures of sunsets and catches of fish on Facebook from those who took the advice of financial planners and coaches like me and are living the good ole life in retirement.

We can't live happy lives mentally or physically if we are worried about money and struggling from paycheck to paycheck. If you need some help to get to your place of financial wellness and are willing to seriously look inward and put forth the necessary work in your financial world, contact me at wealthdiva32@gmail.com and you too can experience *Ohhmazing Wellness* in the financial arena!

Conclusion

My prayer is that you have enjoyed reading all the chapters and found inspiration, guidance, and tips from each co-author as we shared our personal stories with you. I pray you are now better equipped with additional knowledge and understanding to take care of yourself through the integrative wellness process from the eight highlighted areas of self-care. I also pray that the pictures shown of all of us as co-authors gave you a connection to not only read our words but feel our voices and connect with our souls as we shared the common theme for you to shift your vision to create the healthy and happy lifestyle you deserve! Remember that self-care is a way to nurture the body, mind, and soul with the goal of having optimal health in each of these areas. What this might mean depends on your beliefs and lifestyle choices. Your self-care methods might be different from these...yet each of us is doing the very things that bring us health, vitality, success, and satisfaction. Also remember that self-care is important because when we are at our optimal health, we have the energy and stamina to shift our vision and create the healthy and happy lifestyle we deserve!

Do you have certain daily practices that you engage in to keep your mind, body, and soul nourished, well rested and feeling positive as often as possible? In my honesty, one of my greatest challenges to this day is to stay committed to a self-care plan. My plan includes drinking water equal to half my body weight in ounces each day, getting enough sleep for my body type, eating a whole foods plant-based diet, practicing yoga daily, and of course, taking time to nourish my spirit and engaging in the other areas of self-care written about in this book. What does your wellness/self-care plan look like?

CALL TO ACTION!

Connect with us!

Are you ready for a place of endless possibilities—where health and wellness allow you to soar? Are you ready to stretch your limits, lift your spirit, and live every day with vitality and joy? Are you committed to learning the tools and tips to nourish your body, mind, and soul to live a healthy and happy lifestyle? Want to connect with other women from across the globe who share common interests in integrative wellness in the following eight areas:

- Spa and beauty
- Fitness and movement
- Food and nutrition
- Mind and spirit
- Health and holistic healing
- Career and entrepreneurship
- Relationships
- Financial

Gain the knowledge and learn the proper tools and tips for shifting your vision and creating the healthy and happy lifestyle you deserve! Join all of us at www.ohhmazingwellness.com

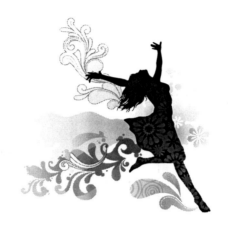

The End

CPSIA information can be obtained
at www.ICGtesting.com
Printed in the USA
FFOW05n2240061114

9 780992 987633